When race counts

The morality of racial preference in
Britain and America

John Edwards

London and New York

First published 1995
by Routledge
11 New Fetter Lane, London EC4P 4EE

Simultaneously published in the USA and Canada
by Routledge
29 West 35th Street, New York, NY 10001

© 1995 John Edwards

Typeset in Baskerville by
Ponting–Green Publishing Services, Chesham, Bucks

Printed and bound in Great Britain by
Biddles Ltd, Guildford and King's Lynn

British Library Cataloguing in Publication Data
A catalogue record for this book is available from the
British Library.

Library of Congress Cataloging in Publication Data
A catalogue record for this book has been requested

ISBN   0–415–07292–1 (hbk)
ISBN   0–415–07293–X (pbk)

When race counts

When Race Counts investigates the use of race-conscious practices in social policy in Britain and America. It questions the distinction between affirmative action and preferential treatment, and evaluates the effectiveness of a range of education and employment policies designed to counteract direct and endemic discrimination against ethnic minorities.

Much of the debate on the condition of racial and ethnic minorities in Britain and America is conducted from entrenched ideological and racial positions. This book aims to break down this unproductive dialogue. The starting point of the analysis in *When Race Counts* is the uncontested deprivation of some ethnic minority groups in many areas of social and economic life, particularly in employment. Given the under-representation of minorities in managerial, professional and other high status professions, the author investigates what action might successfully remedy the situation.

The book uses both empirical and moral analyses to examine the controversial dilemma of whether and in what circumstances preferential treatment may be used as a means of improving the condition of minority groups. John Edwards looks at the justifications for overriding the merit principle, and where the costs and benefits of this lie, arguing that the merit principle is in itself so flawed that no great damage would be done to justice if it were to be overridden for a period by the use of tailored preference policies.

John Edwards is Reader in Social Policy at Royal Holloway, University of London. His previous books include *Positive Discrimination, Social Justice and Social Policy* and *The Enterprise Culture and the Inner City*, both published by Routledge.

For Amy and Bridget

Contents

Illustrations

Foreword

Following the publication of my last excursion into matters of race and positive discrimination, I was urged to write a book on moral discourse in a multi-racial, multicultural society. It was an attractive idea but that book did not get written. This one took over. The same sense of curiosity that led me to embark on that other book however also informs the present one. This curiosity stems in part from a recognition that intuition seems to be a poor guide in matters of racial or ethnic or religious or cultural difference. Preferring people in employment and education just because of their race seems intuitively wrong. So why does it happen and what damage does it do (if any)? And is it any more offensive morally speaking than the old piety of 'merit'? And what if baseline perceptions about what is morally important differ between groups in society?

The focus of the research on which this book is based is those related groups of practices called positive action or affirmative action or positive discrimination or preferential treatment. But the questions that these practices raise go much wider than their immediate impact and this is, therefore, a book both about policy practices and what is morally at issue when we take race into account. Research on affirmative action and preferential treatment on grounds of race was conducted in Great Britain and the United States and on grounds of religious adherence in Northern Ireland. It had been the intention that practice in all three countries would be contained within the compass of the same book, but the volume of material and the complexity of pursuing the arguments through the experience of all three countries proved too much and the story of affirmative action in Northern Ireland forms the basis of another publication.

This book is part empirical and part theoretical (or at least deliberative). The empirical material in Britain and America serves two main purposes. First, it details the nature of affirmative action practices in pursuit of equality of opportunity in employment in both public and private sectors in the two counties, and, of particular relevance to the subsequent discussion, the extent to which these practices shade into preferential treatment. Second, where available data permit, an evaluation of the success of these practices in increasing minority representation is made.

The deliberative content is concerned, amongst many other things, with the morality of preferential treatment. I hope I have been able to make clear why I have been persuaded to the view that preference practice is not entirely morally mischievous – partly as a result of the empirical evidence (particularly from America) and partly from a reappraisal of the nature of merit and the merit principle.

I concluded an earlier work with a (tentative) assertion that positive discrimination was morally unjustified. I have changed my mind. In the field of race research, where knowledge is more often determined from entrenched positions, this must be a unique occurrence.

John Edwards, St Jean D'Aulps

Acknowledgements

Two institutions provided a temporary home during research for this book. I was able to spend a sabbatical year at the Centre for Research in Ethnic Relations at Warwick University and am grateful to friends and colleagues there for support. In particular I would like to thank Malcolm Cross, who was instrumental in arranging my stay.

Tim Barnekov of the College of Urban Affairs and Public Policy at the University of Delaware arranged for my residence there and provided me with a home. I own much to him and to his colleagues at CUAPP.

Thanks are also due to my colleagues in the Department of Social Policy at Royal Holloway College, University of London, for support and stimulation.

Many other people have contributed to this book who must remain anonymous – but in particular those respondents in Britain and America who willingly gave of their time to talk to me and to provide me with data. I learned a great deal from them. What is between these pages seems poor repayment.

The fieldwork for the research was made possible by Economic and Social Research Council grant number R000231148.

The latter part of the book was written under adverse circumstances. I have my wife to thank for having been able to complete it at all.

1   When race counts

We are right to be wary of policies that take explicit account of race. By
such policies we mean those that treat people of different racial groups
differently, and which do so by intent. Too many policies that do this
have been instruments for repression. Their legacy is an unhappy one
and tells us that whatever the ostensible purposes of such policies, there
is a grave danger if race, and indeed religion, are allowed to count, that
once-benign purposes may turn malignant. But present inequalities
between groups that are an inheritance from past harm done by some
groups to others may never be righted by policies that take *no* account
of race. In other words, to put right the wrongs of the past it may be
necessary once more to let race count. Equal treatment now may not
(and probably will not) abolish present inequalities that are the legacy
of past unequal treatment, and it may be necessary, in order to achieve
a greater inter-group equality, to treat different groups differently – in
other words, to let race count.

If, therefore, employment, education, housing and health policies
(to name only a few) are to be sensitive to people's race or ethnic
background, in order to establish a greater inter-group equality, we
need to ask how far we are justified in giving special help or preference
to disadvantaged groups, because to do so appears to promote just
those sorts of policy of which we ought to be wary. This is the dilemma
of affirmative action and preferential treatment practices. Both types
of practice are, within the contexts in which they are used, race-
conscious,[1] and preferential treatment more so than affirmative action,
though, as we shall see, they are not discrete practices but rather the
two ends of a continuum. And because of their race-centredness, both
types of practice have been the subject of much debate. For some, they
are the only way to achieve equality and equity between groups; for
others their use will serve only to harden and crystallise racial divisions
in society. For those who take the latter view, practices towards the
preferential treatment end of the continuum are manifestly unjust
because they must entail (in the area of employment with which we
shall primarily be concerned) the hiring or promotion of a less well

qualified minority (or target) group member in preference to a better qualified majority group member, in an effort to reduce minority group under-representation in the workforce (or a particular part of it). In short, putting right the wrongs of the past requires that we create more wrongs by overriding the merit principle of 'the best person for the job' which must be the foundation of all good employment practice. Or so orthodox practice would have it. We shall see, however, that matters are more complex than this simple argument allows, and 'merit' turns out to be a rather less pristine principle than is often thought. There is, in consequence, scope for a defence of policies of preference as well as of affirmative action.

Virtually all public policy (and private policy in the employment field) is supposedly indifferent to the race of the people it affects. We do not, on the whole, have different pensions or housing or employment or health policies for people of different races. If we did, we would rightly be wary of their motives.[2] Social policies and practices that do focus differentially on racial groups, therefore, will inevitably be subject to particular scrutiny. Our concern in this study is with such groups and the practices which focus upon them. The groups that we are concerned with are racial and ethnic groups, that all have in common a relatively deprived status in employment, housing, income, education and a number of other areas when compared with the majority.[3] It is this relative deprivation of whole groups, identifiable by race or religion, that calls forth *group*-based practices. And this is what makes affirmative action and preferential treatment distinctive and in need of closer moral scrutiny. The beneficiaries of orthodox social policies, if they are defined in group terms at all, are so classified on the basis of morally relevant group characteristics such as need, or having special needs or on criteria of desert or merit (see Edwards 1987: Chapter 3). There is no prima-facie reason, on the other hand, why social and public policy should treat people differently on the basis of morally irrelevant criteria such as race, and when they do there must be good reasons why they do. This requirement lies at the heart of the present study.

Conventional social policies – that is, policies that take no account of race – appear to have been relatively ineffective at reducing inequalities between minority and majority groups.[4] Now if it were just a matter of minority groups having average levels of needs that were greater than the average levels of needs in the majority group, and if conventional policies allocated resources in proportion to need, then there is no obvious reason why they should not be effective in reducing group inequalities. But the fact that such inequalities persist is in some measure due to past and continuing discrimination of a variety of types and it is of this that conventional policies fail to take account. Discrimination may be inducing needs as fast as conventional policies meet them. We do, of course, recognise direct discrimination against the individual by another or by an institution and there is legislation in many countries that makes such discrimination on the basis of race or religion (and of other factors) a criminal act. But it is not primarily this kind of discrimination that contributes to the relative deprivations of whole groups. Where discrimination is contributory to group social and economic inequalities, it is more likely to be indirect, institutional, often unintended, sometimes unrecognised and endemic. It is this sort of discrimination and its effects that go largely untouched by either social policy or anti-discrimination legislation. Neither is orthodox social policy very sensitive to the multiplicity of factors that contribute to inequalities between groups – of which discrimination in its variety of forms is but one. Hence the need for – or at least the attraction of – race- and religion-conscious policies that are more likely to take account of those factors, peculiar to certain groups, that contribute to their deprivation relative to the majority (and to each other).

The first step onto the continuum of practices that reaches from affirmative action to preferential treatment comes with the recognition of the part that systemic discrimination plays in creating and replicating the relative deprivation of some groups by denying access to goods and services, and by compromising opportunities that ought to be equal to those of majority group members. If, therefore, members of particular minority groups are under-represented in certain occupations or positions, or if they are concentrated in the worst quality housing or over-represented amongst the poor, then this may be seen to be the result of inequality of opportunities in education and employment and of policies which *de facto* discriminate against them. Such a diagnosis then leads to the promotion of practices designed to remove discriminatory barriers to opportunities and goods and services. Practices of this kind we call affirmative action, though 'barrier removal' is not their entirety: there is more to affirmative action than that. Nonetheless, the removal of discriminatory barriers to equality of opportunities with others and to the provision of goods and services commensurate in quality and quantity with the relative needs of minority and majority groups can be seen as the first step away from policies that are blind to race and religion. Affirmative action as barrier removal must, by its very nature, take account of them, though it may be made to appear neutral (and neutralising) in intention and effects. Even more so is this the case when affirmative action develops from barrier removal (such as eliminating discriminatory personnel practices) towards activity that tries to compensate for discrimination, such as concentrating recruiting efforts in minority schools or areas, or advertising posts in the minority press.

Such practices as these, though race-conscious, may be defended in the employment realm at least on the grounds that although special efforts are made to recruit more minority candidates for job or post vacancies, race plays no part in the selection process. The successful candidate will be the best person for the job irrespective of race.

Our intuitive notions of justice would be less satisfied, however, if, in the provision of goods and services such as housing, education, income support or health, we were to give additional resources to minority groups, even if this were to be defended on the grounds of higher average levels of need among such groups. The difference between this and the case of education is that in the latter affirmative action is attempting only to equalise opportunities whilst in the former it is exercising real preference to minorities (which *would* be justified if all minority group members had greater needs than all majority group members – a situation only very rarely to be found).

The moral dilemmas of race-conscious practices increase the further we move along the continuum from the sorts of affirmative action described above towards what has been characterised as preferential treatment, a discussion of which takes up much of the latter part of this study. It is here that practices appear to breach the canons of justice (or, at least, fairness) by overriding the principle of merit.

Our purpose is not primarily either to promote or to detract from affirmative action or preferential treatment but rather to approach these important areas of public policy with a sense of curiosity. The arguments for and against race-conscious policies, when they are not part of a rhetorical crusade, are complex and, it seems to me, a close-run thing. The arguments must necessarily proceed on a number of fronts, principally the moral, the practical and the pragmatic, but all these are inter-connected and a large part of our task will be to counterbalance arguments on each front. What may in practice and pragmatically be successful may, on the other hand, prove morally unacceptable. Practices that are morally unobjectionable may simply not work and so on.

In an attempt to give substance to our arguments, but also as a means of mapping out current affirmative action and preferential treatment practices, we have looked at examples of practice in two countries – Great Britain and the United States. The race-conscious practices of public and private sector agencies recounted here are not intended to be representative of all current practice in these two countries, but rather they are illustrative of the sorts of practice that are current, and of the sorts of results that are being obtained in terms of minority group representation in employment and education. Neither is the choice of countries intended to be representative of race- and religion-conscious practice in general. The United States selects itself as the country where race-conscious practices are most extensive and widely used and where debate about them is most finely developed. The American experience must be the touchstone against which practice elsewhere should be tested. Great Britain, on the other hand, was selected simply because it is home territory and provides a valuable comparison in terms of race-conscious policy with the United States.

But this is not, strictly speaking, a comparative study. We make no attempt at systematic comparisons of practice or results between the two countries. Rather, experience in one country is used to illustrate that in the other and arguments developed in one are used in analyses of the other.

Policies and practices that differentiate between people on the basis of their race, whether in the public or private sectors, must inevitably be contentious, even though their purposes are benign towards those groups that appear to be relatively disadvantaged. It is not just that history warns us of the dangers, it is more pragmatically that such practices are not costless and that majority group members who bear the costs (the white candidate who does not get the job because it had to go to a black candidate under a preference quota) don't see why they should because *they* are not responsible for the relative deprivations of the minority. It is not surprising, therefore, that promoting race-conscious practices is not an attractive position for any serious political party to adopt. Indeed, both countries proscribe preferential treatment. But it is practised nonetheless in varying degrees – and extensively so in the United States. It must be one of our central concerns, therefore, to explain why contentious and (to many) unpopular practices are pursued, often with vigour, not only by local governments and universities, which may be assumed to carry in some measure a social welfare mandate, but by private sector agencies also.

This then is the ground that we shall tread. It is a wide panorama but always at its centre will be the questions of when, and under what circumstances, and for what reasons, will race-conscious practices be justified as instruments of public policy.

2 The nature and varieties of affirmative action

Affirmative, or positive, action practices are, in theory at least, conceptually and morally distinct from both preferential treatment (positive discrimination) on the one hand, and ordinary practice on the other. If they were not, then much of the debate about race-conscious practice that has exercised practitioners, commentators, the legislature and the judiciary in the United States, the United Kingdom and elsewhere would be otiose. The fact is that race-conscious practices *are* different if only because they appear to contradict the philosophy of non-discrimination that underlies almost all policy and which is itself, albeit inadequately, underpinned by statute or constitution, or both, in the US and Great Britain.

A part of our task will be to examine when, and under what circumstances, practices that take race into account are permissible both morally and statutorily. Another part will be to evaluate the success of such practices when they are used. A prerequisite of both tasks, and a number of others that we shall undertake along the way, must be a specification of affirmative action that identifies it as a set of discrete practices and which distinguishes it both from preferential treatment and from 'ordinary' race-blind practice. Two potential sources of confusion must first be clarified however. When we speak of affirmative action (and preferential treatment) as race-conscious practice,[1] we do not mean to imply that all such policies or practices constitute affirmative action. Special dispensations in respect of clothing or holiday allowances or cultural needs (see Commission for Racial Equality 1980, 1984) or provision for race as a genuine occupational qualification (see Home Office 1977) or racially-biased immigration policies are not affirmative action. The term 'affirmative action' will be confined to policies and practices in areas where policy is conventionally colour-blind and where there is no prima-facie moral or functional reason for believing that race is relevant to policy intent or output.

The second source of potential confusion lies in the implicit assertion above that affirmative action can be distinguished from preferential treatment. There is a great deal of misuse of the two terms (but especially of their British counterparts 'positive action' and 'positive discrimination'), either wilful or as a result of ignorance or confusion, that would suggest that they are not clearly distinguishable – or at least not easily so. More importantly, informed debate in the US suggests that the borderline between affirmative action and preferential treatment is far from distinctly drawn (see for example Fullinwider 1986, Ruzicho 1980, Abram 1986, Kennedy 1986, Steele 1990a). Whilst the inconsistent use of the two terms in Britain (and to a lesser extent in America) owes less to any real conceptual difficulty in distinguishing between them than to a want of critical analysis, it remains true that though a theoretical dividing line does exist, in practice there is only a blurred division between affirmative action and preferential treatment and they are more usefully conceived of as two points on a continuum. That does not mean, however, that as ideal types the two ideas are indistinguishable. We shall be concerned with both concepts and, where it is necessary to distinguish between the two, the use of terminology will reflect this.

STARTING POINT: RACIAL INEQUALITIES

We wish to avoid characterising affirmative action by its colloquial usage. That would simply be to build into our analysis the errors and inconsistencies that we seek to avoid. What subsequent paragraphs seek to do therefore is to derive a distinct meaning for affirmative action from first principles. The derivation will proceed in a number of sequential stages, the first of which is to identify the perceived reasons why some form of action like affirmative action is deemed to be desirable or necessary. (The reason for seeming to restate the blindingly obvious is that we are sometimes blinded by the obvious.)

The motive force behind race-focused affirmative action is the perceived under-representation or under-utilisation of the affected groups in certain occupations, professions, statuses and positions and their over-representation among the unemployed. Second, there is the perceived over-representation of such groups among those suffering a range of social and economic disadvantages or their unique exposure to a more compounded form of deprivation (usually called racial disadvantage) (see House of Commons 1981, Smith 1977, Benyon and Solomos 1987, Brown 1984).[2]

There will be more to say subsequently about the nature and extent of the under-representation of minority groups in occupations, professions and positions, but for the purpose of the present argument it is enough to take these as a 'given'. It should be noted, however, that the picture that emerges will be very different depending on whether what we measure is 'under-representation' or 'under-utilisation' (the latter being a term used by the Office of Federal Contract Compliance

Programs in the US to describe a part of its Affirmative Action Programs). Under-representation is usually taken to mean a comparison between the representation of a minority group in an occupation or position and its representation in the labour force as a whole – or sometimes, more crudely, its representation in the population as a whole. Under-utilisation on the other hand gives a comparison between representation in an occupation, position, establishment, etc. and the *availability* of members of the affected group. Availability is measured by eight factors and produces a figure that represents the numbers who might be available and qualified for the relevant position or status (see Cooper 1987: Chapter 4, United States Code of Federal Regulations 1989: Title 41, Chapter 60–2.11). Under-utilisation therefore, gives a *more* accurate (though far from accurate) picture of the extent to which a company or establishment is *discriminating*, but it takes little account of the effects of *past* discrimination and present *disadvantage* that will have depressed the numbers of the affected group who are currently suitably qualified for the position.

Under-representation and under-utilisation, therefore, measure different things and will produce different results, but a showing on either that fewer minority group members are in place than would be expected provides prima-facie evidence of the operation of discrimination or disadvantage or (*but not necessarily*) both.

The next, and subsequent, stages of our derivation of affirmative action will concentrate on under-representation and under-utilisation as the starting point rather than evidence of over-representation in disadvantage, but the latter will necessarily enter our discussion when we draw in the idea of equality of opportunity.

REASONS FOR UNDER-REPRESENTATION AND UNDER-UTILISATION

The reasons for the under-representation and under-utilisation of affected minorities will differ, at least in their relative balance as between the two measures. Subsequent analysis will take account of this but for the moment we can combine the two measures and will refer to both as under-representation. Conceptually, there appear to be two dominant reasons why members of affected groups are less in evidence in some occupations and positions[3] than might be expected from their representation in the labour force, the population as a whole, or from their 'availability'.

✳ The first is that members of affected groups do not have equality of opportunity to compete for and obtain desired positions and statuses. Whether this amounts to a multiplicity of *individual* inequalities of opportunity or to something that we might call *group* inequality of opportunity is something that will have to be clarified before we can arrive at a specification of affirmative action.

The second reason may lie in the relatively greater, or different, social and economic disadvantages from which minorities suffer and which we identified in the previous section as being one cause of initial concern.

These two dominant reasons are not, of course, mutually exclusive, either conceptually or empirically. Some aspects of disadvantage are counted-in as components of lack of equality of opportunity on some interpretations of that concept (see Williams 1962, Sher 1977, Standing Advisory Commission on Human Rights 1987: 43, Rawls 1972: 83–90, Raphael 1976: 187–90, Guttman 1980: 107–13). Otherwise they may be treated as acting independently of opportunity, equality of which is then seen to be a function only of discriminatory barriers. This, however, is a very limited notion of equality of opportunity, and our purpose is better served by counting disadvantage (in whatever form) as constituent of the factors that create less than equality of opportunity.

We can say therefore that the dominant reason for the under-representation of minorities is lack of equality of opportunity, where this consists of discriminatory barriers (either direct or indirect, intentional or unintentional), greater relative disadvantage (interpreted as higher proportions of minority group members suffering from disadvantage, or minority groups on the whole suffering higher levels of disadvantage, or both), different forms of disadvantage – and hence special need – or a compounding of disadvantages that would enable us to speak of racial disadvantage as a specific type of a more generic concept. This will suffice for the moment but our formulation of 'disadvantage' is less than adequate and will require some tidying up before we evaluate the effectiveness of policies. It leaves unanswered, for example, the question of whether such phenomena as 'unfamiliarity', cultural differences, community mores and family expectations and demands are aspects of disadvantage. That they have an effect on the ability of minority group members to compete in the merit system, on the range of choices open to them and (particularly in the case of some minority women) the extent to which pursuit of a career can be a priority seems evident. They do, nonetheless, appear to fall into a different category to social and economic disadvantages, if only because some at least are not entirely unwanted by some (and possibly many) members of the minority group.

One final, and related, caveat must be entered to the arguments in this section. It is simply this: that lack of equal opportunity, even in its widest interpretation, does not fully account for the under-representation of minority group members. There is a very murky and as yet almost unresearched set of factors that will affect people's employment paths. These we may call choices or preferences or more accurately *unconstrained* choices or preferences. What we shall need to discover about these is the extent to which systematically different choices are made by different groups in a multicultural society such as would lead us to expect systematic differences of distribution in the employment field even given complete equality of opportunity. For the moment, however, it is enough to record that it seems unlikely that the eradication of inequality of opportunity would lead to equality of representation both horizontal and vertical across the entire employment (and non-employment) spectrum.

REASONS FOR INEQUALITY OF OPPORTUNITY

Outlining the reasons for the lack of equality of opportunity that was identified above requires that we should specify the components of equal opportunity (as opposed to alternative interpretations of the concept). Leaving aside the grey areas of constrained choice or preference, there are at least four in number:[4]

- biological or genetic endowments (see Rosenberg 1987); these will partly determine future activities, abilities to compete and so forth of all participants in the employment system, but so far as the relative *group* inequality of opportunity of minorities is concerned, what is of relevance here is the sets of biological endowments of members of minority groups *vis-à-vis* members of the majority;
- non-biological characteristics and qualities of minority group members *vis-à-vis* the majority such as preparedness or willingness to make efforts and sacrifices, energy, determination and so on (there is no identifiable dividing line between these and biological endowments);
- disadvantage which may be more extensive or quantitatively greater or qualitatively different for minority groups;
- direct and indirect discrimination which by definition is peculiar to minority groups (though discrimination in other forms may affect other groups in society).

The first three of these (along with a number of other factors of less importance) will, to the extent that they are possessed or not, affect the social and economic life-chances of *all* members of society. The fourth will be an additional factor affecting only members of groups that suffer discrimination. But insofar as equality of opportunity for *groups* as opposed to *individuals* is concerned,[5] the first two components are of dubious utility. That biological endowments differ as between different racial and ethnic groups is self-evident. That any of these differences *per se* is such as to affect performance in the employment domain, or that any individual biological attribute that might affect performance differs systematically between groups, is neither self-evident nor revealed by any empirical scrutiny. There are no grounds for saying,

therefore, that individual biological endowments are in any way contributive to *group* inequality of opportunity. (They are, of course, highly
relevant to individual opportunity or, more pertinently, to individual
chances if opportunity is interpreted to mean opportunity to fulfil
individual *potential* rather than to reach a given status or position
(see Edwards 1990a).)

The same may be said of non-biological attributes, though the terrain
here is rougher and strewn with obstacles, and there is sufficient
evidence to make the contention less than self-evident. (This component would at least have to be entertained, for example, in any
comprehensive explanation of the relative academic, occupational and
economic success of the Jewish and Chinese populations of America
(see Killian 1990, Hacker 1989).) There is little or nothing to be gained
for present purposes however from pursuing this line of argument and
our attention should focus on the last two components.

Insofar, therefore, as *group* inequality of opportunity is concerned,
we can say that the two main contributory factors are discrimination
and disadvantage and, to the extent that both are treated as components of unequal opportunity, they are best characterised as unfair
barriers to exploiting opportunities and as relative disadvantages at
getting over fair hurdles in the way to exploiting opportunities respectively. An example of the first might be employment tests that are
not neutral as between racial and religious groups, and of the second,
relative lack of genuine qualifications for positions.

A REMEDIAL STRATEGY

In the most general of terms what would be required to remedy the
situation described in the foregoing paragraphs would be action of
some sort to remove both direct and indirect discrimination for affected
groups and alleviate the greater or distinctive disadvantages that they
suffer. There are, of course, a variety of ways in which (and degrees to
which) both of these could be done. Any such practice, however, would
have at least one distinctive characteristic – it would operate in respect
of the affected group(s) and not in respect of individuals. It would, in
short, be a *group* practice and the groups at which it was targeted would
be arbitrarily defined from a moral point of view. One such type of
practice we may call positive or affirmative action. (Another, yet to be
distinguished, would be preferential treatment.)

A practice or set of practices to alleviate discrimination and disadvantage will need, in relation to the former, because discrimination is
by definition group-specific,[6] to be directed at removing practices or
actions which are intentionally or unintentionally discriminatory in
respect of *the group*; barriers to individual equality of opportunity would
not be part of such practice. Alleviating disadvantages that are experi-

enced to a greater degree by, or are of a different kind for, an affected group creates rather more conceptual and moral puzzles and it is a consideration of these that will lead us to a clearer specification of the moral standing of affirmative action, including its relation to preferential treatment.

Disadvantage, in its generic sense, is not confined to minority ethnic groups; as I have noted elsewhere, the majority of the deprived and disadvantaged, in Great Britain at least, are white (Edwards 1987: 201). What then are the moral grounds for introducing group-based policies to relieve disadvantage (that is, ones the purpose of which is not to distribute resources in proportion to the degree of individual disadvantage or need but to benefit differentially a group, membership of which is not defined by degree of need or disadvantage but by the morally arbitrary criterion of race) when the majority of the disadvantaged are not members of the group and similar policies are not implemented in respect of them? We have already canvassed three possible reasons and we must now look at these to see if they prescribe a distinctive and discrete practice we may call 'positive action'. They are claims that (a) higher proportions of the membership of affected groups are disadvantaged than is the case for the non-minority; (b) the affected group as a whole suffers higher levels of disadvantage than does the majority; and (c) the affected group suffers from distinctive types of disadvantage which may be called racial disadvantage.

That the first of these is true in respect of some aspects of disadvantage is lent support by empirical evidence, though the nature and extent of the disadvantage does vary from one group to another (see Brown 1984, Steele 1990b).

The inference that might be drawn from this is that were group remedial practices to be adopted then they ought to be specific to particular groups and should not apply to all minority racial groups in an undifferentiated way. However, to the extent that it is true that higher proportions of (some) minority groups suffer from disadvantage, the adoption of a group practice to alleviate the disadvantage will not necessarily identify for us a morally distinctive practice. As has been argued elsewhere (Edwards 1987: 42–55, Miller 1976, Feinberg 1973, Campbell 1988), a specification of just distributions requires that morally relevant material principles of formal justice (i.e. those things that do justify us in distributing social goods and resources differentially between people) be distinguished from the morally arbitrary characteristics of people which do not justify different treatment or differential distributions. Morally relevant criteria for just distributions turn out to be few in number and varied in composition depending on your chosen philosopher,[7] but there is consensus on a central core which includes rights, needs and desert. Examples of criteria (or human characteristics) which are arbitrary from a moral point of view in respect of how people should be treated or distributions made (i.e. which do *not* justify different treatment or distributions) would be race, religious adherence, skin colour, sex, eye or hair colour and so on.[8] Since affirmative action, in the way we have characterised it so far, identifies its beneficiaries by their race or ethnicity therefore, it is prima facie an unjust practice (and hence, morally at least, discrete). However, the argument from greater incidence of disadvantage turns the morally arbitrary criteria of race or ethnicity into proxy measures of social need and hence into morally relevant criteria. In short, the argument would be that since greater proportions of minority group members than of majority group members suffer from disadvantage, adopting practices that take minority group members as their target is really an alternative and possibly administratively more efficient way of meeting needs and can be justified on these grounds. Affirmative action, though apparently distinctive because it uses morally arbitrary criteria to select bene-ficiaries, then becomes indistinguishable other than administratively from other need-meeting practices (which are usually individual rather than group-based).

Similar arguments will apply in respect of the claim that overall levels of disadvantage are greater for minority than for majority groups, though empirically this would be more difficult to demonstrate, requir-ing as it would some quantitative average levels of disadvantage for different groups on a range of disadvantages or deprivations. None-theless, on the assumption that this could be done and the appropriate results achieved, the same argument could be turned to effect – that using race as the group-identifying criterion would be simply to use it as a proxy for need groups.

The claim that *racial* disadvantage was the operative barrier to equality of opportunity raises somewhat different problems for justice arguments. Racial disadvantage, as we have noted, is a peculiar type of disadvantage in which deprivations that are shared with the majority are compounded by race-specific disadvantages and (on some accounts) by negative discrimination. To the extent that racial disadvantage is seen as a special need then it must compete with the needs of other special need groups. The difficulty with this, however, is that other special need groups are identified by a morally relevant criterion (their particular special need) whereas racial groups are definitionally identified by a morally arbitrary criterion – race.

Governments have trod warily over this ground when they have dealt with race matters but we can usefully bring this brief excursion into special needs and racial disadvantage to an end by citing the British government's response to the Home Affairs Committee Report on racial disadvantage. This tip-toed round the question of how to justify meeting the special needs of minorities but not the different (and special?) needs of non-minority group members. And by equating the special needs of minority groups with those of 'other groups in special need', it entirely missed the moral crux of the matter – that meeting the needs of a morally arbitrarily defined group requires special justification in a way that meeting the needs of special need groups (the elderly, the handicapped, children at risk) does not. This is what the government said on the question of the needs of ethnic minorities:

> Where the needs of the ethnic minorities are different from or greater than those of the majority population, special measures may be called for (*as they are for other groups in special need*) . . . concern is frequently expressed that to follow this course would be to give members of the ethnic minority communities an unfair advantage over the majority population. The Government accepts that measures that had this effect would be undesirable. . . . The Government believes, however, that if the aim of equality of opportunity for all members of society is to be achieved, special help will often be needed for those who start from a position of comparative disadvantage. The ethnic minorities are one group [sic] for whom there is a need to redress existing imbalances.
>
> (House of Commons, 1982, emphasis added)

This masterpiece of insipidity bears all the right sentiments (it could equally well have come from an Anglican prelate) and carries minimal conviction. It does, nonetheless, attempt to square the circle. There is recognition of the danger of white reaction, the attempt to equate ethnic minorities with special need groups, the rejection of advantageous treatment, the appeal to equality of opportunity for all – and then the 'justifier' – that ethnic minorities start from 'comparative disadvantage' and this requires that we 'redress . . . imbalances'. (It always sounds so *reasonable* and so easy to redress imbalances.) We are justified therefore in meeting the *special* needs of morally arbitrarily defined groups because they turn out to be *greater* needs (hence the 'comparative disadvantage' and the 'imbalance'). And so, on this rendering at least, the special needs argument becomes subsumed within the greater needs argument we have aired above, and affirmative action for minority groups is simply a more convenient way of fulfilling the needs principle.

There are logical objections to this line of argument. It works as a justifier for affirmative action only under two conditions. The first is that the special needs are in addition to that level of needs which the most needy in the majority population have – that is, the minority groups have the same levels of need as those of majority group members in need *plus* the special needs. The second (alternative) condition is that the sum of the ordinary and special needs of minorities is such as to put them in a position of having greater needs than those in the majority whose level of need would justify the allocation of resources. The difficulty here is that special needs, because they are special, cannot be quantified on some monotonic scale along with 'ordinary' needs.

The argument from special needs therefore requires a good deal more care in its application than the bland essay we have quoted. There are obvious examples of special or different needs which some ethnic minority group members have which constitute a formidable barrier to equality of opportunity – poor grasp of the English language would be one – and which the promotion of *equality* of opportunity would require be met. But that having special needs *per se* (whatever they may be) justifies that these needs be met by a group practice aimed at a morally arbitrarily defined group – that is, independently of and outside the needs principle, and hence potentially in preference to others not in the group who may have great needs but not ones that are special – remains less than convincing.

What we have so far, therefore, is a strategy which may be positive action or positive discrimination which is distinctive because, unlike other social policies, it takes a morally arbitrarily defined group as its target. It does this because of the evidence of under-representation of minority group members in some positions and statuses and because of the assumed reasons for this under-representation. And because the target group is a morally arbitrary one, the practice is prima facie unjust. It can (so the argument goes) be justified by showing that the pattern of needs and disadvantages from which the group suffers (and which limits its opportunities) is such that the needs principle would not be overridden by meeting needs on the group basis. The moral arbitrariness of the group is made morally relevant by the greater or additional or (less convincingly) the special needs that it has compared with the majority. Justice, via the needs principle, will not be compromised, because any preference that might be given will be preference for the most needy. These arguments have been well rehearsed, particularly in the American literature (see in particular the exchanges in *Analysis* over the period 1972–75: Cowan 1972, Nickel 1972, 1973, Bayles 1973b, Nunn 1973, Shiner 1973, Silvestri 1973, Taylor 1973, Goldman 1975). Ultimately, however, the substitutability of morally relevant for morally arbitrary criteria must turn upon an empirical estimation of the degree of correlation between the distribution of need or disadvantage and of minority groups in the population, unless a stronger case can be made for special needs being an adequate justifier in themselves. The degree of correlation will vary from one country to another of course, and hence the strength of the case for justifying group practices by the substitution of morally relevant criteria.

A MORAL SPECIFICATION OF AFFIRMATIVE ACTION

Notwithstanding the arguments cited above for a justifying of what appears prima facie to be an unjust practice, affirmative action (as we have so far called it) remains distinctive insofar as it is a group-based practice and that the beneficiary groups are defined by morally arbitrary criteria. This in itself has distributive implications for the justifying arguments. Group-based practices of the kind we have been discussing are, by their very nature, indifferent to distributions *within* the affected groups. It has long been a contention of opponents of affirmative action and preferential treatment in the United States, for example, that insofar as the motivating force for such practices is compensation for past harm (discrimination),[9] they are poor mechanisms for ensuring that the most harmed gain the most benefit (and indeed, that the worst perpetrators of discrimination bear the heaviest costs). And there is, it must be said, some evidence to support this in that the main beneficiaries of affirmative action and preference have been middle-class blacks and Hispanics (see, for example, Abram 1986, Steele 1990a, Potomac Institute 1984, Carter 1991 and Belz 1991).

The same argument applies in respect of meeting needs to alleviate disadvantage. There can be no guarantee that the main beneficiaries of (for example) training programmes or outreach efforts, or validated tests or race awareness programmes are just those who have suffered the most disadvantage or faced the most pernicious discriminatory barriers. It may of course be argued that at the level of group practice this is inevitable and what we are concerned with is precisely the improvement of the condition of the group as a whole. We shall have much more to say about this in subsequent chapters. For the moment it is enough to note that the very fact of being a group-based practice, where the beneficiary groups are identified by morally arbitrary criteria, makes affirmative action (and cognate practices) morally distinctive. (And whether the moral arbitrariness of the group can then be 'justified' by the claim that it is really a proxy for a morally relevant one becomes, as we have noted, an empirical question.) What may matter in the longer run is whether we (including minority group members) care more about group or individual justice.

It is time to turn our attention to other components of a moral specification of affirmative action and for this it is necessary to distinguish between two characteristics of group practices. The first is the selected target groups; the second, the particular procedures adopted in an affirmative action or preferential treatment programme. This division will better enable us to make at least a conceptual distinction between affirmative action and other forms of race-conscious practice.

Thus far we have identified a group practice designed to reduce first-order discrimination and alleviate deprivation and disadvantage which in varying degrees (and for a variety of reasons) appears to be group-related. This practice we have called, for the sake of convenience, 'affirmative action'. It is now necessary to distinguish within this generic type between 'true' affirmative action and preferential treatment (otherwise known in America as 'reverse discrimination'[10] and in Britain as 'positive discrimination'). Affirmative action and preferential treatment do not differ on the first of the components noted above; the target groups and their moral arbitrariness are the same for both sorts of practice. And it is the moral arbitrariness of the beneficiary groups that makes both practices prima facie unjust. If a distinction is to be made between affirmative action and preferential treatment, it lies in the second component – the particular procedures adopted – and we shall compare the procedures characteristic of both practices in relation both to the removal or overcoming of discrimination and to the alleviation of disadvantage.

Now, it needs to be said that whilst there are conceptual and moral differences between affirmative action and preferential treatment, and we shall have reason throughout this work to pay attention to these differences, it is not our view that affirmative action and preference are best characterised by their moral differences. There is, in practice, no clear dividing line between the two sorts of policy; their moral similarities are probably more significant than their differences and it seems more promising to treat them as two parts of a monotonic continuum. This is the approach we shall adopt. To begin with though we shall clarify such important distinctions as there are between preference policy and affirmative action.

What distinguishes the procedures used by affirmative action and preferential treatment in respect both of discrimination and of disadvantage is the extent to which they conform with what principles of distributive justice would demand, and in pursuing this line of argument it will be necessary briefly to encroach on the substance of later chapters in order at least to identify (if not at this stage fully resolve) an apparent anomaly. The difficulty is this.

The procedures of affirmative action to overcome discrimination or its effects are said in most respects not to override the canons of justice. What is done is, by means of procedures such as outreach, special training, advertising jobs in the ethnic minority press and so on, to bring more minority group members to the interview room. That is all. Thereafter merit and merit alone must decide who is appointed or promoted. Sometimes, as a means of incentives to more robust action and as a measure of progress, goals or targets and associated timetables are set. But, in theory at least, they remain goals, and if they are not met the only consequence will be (again in theory) that efforts of the same kind must be redoubled. Preferential treatment, on the other hand, will use the same procedures but characteristically will set quotas rather than goals. Unmet quotas may carry penalties and their fulfilment will involve appointing or promoting less well qualified minority group members over better qualified majority group members if necessary.[11] In short, preferential treatment overrides the merit principle and *this is usually taken to involve flouting the demands of justice*. And it is primarily for this reason that preferential treatment is deemed to be unacceptable (and illegal).

In the reasoning outlined above a good deal of weight is attached to the merit principle (and to merit) such that it is treated as inviolable. But it is worth reiterating that when governments find it most necessary to acclaim merit, it is normally by way of a warning not to let goals become quotas rather than a castigation of the evils of negative discrimination. Now the anomaly lies in the apparent apodicity with which merit is imbued in these and many similar sentiments. It is hard to see why merit should be treated as though it were a prescriptive principle of justice. Certainly, to allocate jobs on a principle of merit, provided we all accept and agree to the components of this chimeric concept, would seem to be 'fair' (in the sense of playing by the rules of the game), but two considerations at least should give us reason to doubt its deonticity. The first is that we cannot be said to *deserve* much of what constitutes merit (we no more deserve our IQ than our ethnicity), and second what constitutes merit is what is deemed to be functional for job performance, which makes merit a soundly consequential concept not one that it is right (morally speaking) to pursue in and of itself.

To the extent therefore that the difference between affirmative action and preferential treatment hinges on the idea of merit (to override it or not), it is not as morally critical a difference as conventional wisdom would have us believe. It is not the difference between a just and an unjust practice – at least insofar as respect for merit is concerned. Neither is it possible to draw a clear distinction between affirmative action and preferential treatment at the level of practice, as later case studies will demonstrate. More realistically, as already noted, we should see both types of practice as the ends of a continuum of race- or religion-conscious practice. We shall have more to say on this in later chapters.

The second dimension we noted above, on which the procedures of affirmative action and preferential treatment may vary, is in the alleviation of deprivation. Once more, the caveat must be made that it makes more sense to view the two practices as the opposite ends of a continuum rather than as sharply distinguishable, and this is even more the case when we consider the meeting of needs to relieve disadvantage. As in the case of discrimination we can attempt to distinguish affirmative action from preferential treatment by measuring their respective procedures against the commands of justice. The relevant material principle of justice here is of course 'need', and we may assume that insofar as need is morally relevant to distribution, justice will require that we distribute in proportion to it (see Edwards 1987: Chapter 4). Two difficulties then present themselves: one a general problem of need-meeting given any finite level of resources, the other specific to group-related practices.

If needs are defined in any other than an absolute way, they will be endlessly extensionable (Braybrooke 1968, 1987, Edwards 1988). Available resources, on the other hand, given the extent of other demands on governments, are finite. Not all needs can therefore be met and the question of allocating by need becomes one of the distribution of need-meeting itself (see Weale 1978). What needs should be met and to what level of satisfaction, and what needs must perforce go unmet? In practice, in any area of welfare provision this is a pretty haphazard affair and it is often not possible to say whether some people's needs are being met to a degree that necessarily precludes the satisfaction of the equal or greater needs of others. This does not obviate the desirability (to put it no higher) of some guidelines and for present purposes the idea of 'equality of welfare' will prove useful. This has been articulated by Weale (1978: Chapter 5; see also Edwards 1987: Chapter 4) and is in essence an argument that needs be met in proportion to their degree up to a level at which everyone with needs has attained an equal level of welfare.[12] Where that level will be will depend on available resources; it will be below the level at which all needs have been satisfied but it will ensure that all those remaining in need will have had a justifiable quantum of their needs met and that such needs as remain will be equally distributed. What the 'equality of welfare' principle attempts to prevent, therefore, is inequity in the meeting of need.

The second problem arises because we are dealing with group practices. The material principles of justice – and indeed the equality of welfare principle as normally interpreted – take individuals as their datum. Now whilst there is no logical reason why we cannot substitute groups for individuals in either concept, it has to be recognised that comparison of *group* needs and measuring notional equality of welfare as between groups are in practice extremely difficult – and particularly so once we introduce the notion of special needs which cannot be summed on a monotonic scale. Nonetheless, the theoretical substitution of groups for individuals will suffice for the present purpose of finding a diagnostic of the difference between affirmative action and preferential treatment.

A group practice that conformed to the requirements of justice in distribution for need-meeting would be one that allocated resources to different groups[13] in proportion to their different needs until all groups had reached equality of benefit at the point when available resources had been exhausted. All groups would have had their needs met to an equal level of satisfaction. Such a description would characterise affirmative action procedures. Preferential treatment in need-meeting on the other hand would give one or more groups greater resources than would be justified by their degree of need and would, at the expense of other groups, take them beyond notional equality of welfare. Other groups with similar needs would have fewer of their needs met because the preferred group(s) had had more; it would have been an unjust distribution.

Whilst this formulation provides the means to distinguish between affirmative action and preferential treatment when they are used to overcome disadvantage, it is nonetheless fraught with difficulties, only the more salient of which we need point out here. How are the needs of each group to be calculated in a way that will make them comparable? We can of course use some average figure (average unemployment rates for Afro-Caribbeans, Indians, Pakistanis, Bangladeshis, whites) but do we, because we are using group practices, wish entirely to ignore distributions within groups? Will justice be done (to all groups) by treating the white majority as virtually homogeneous? Would even affirmative action, on these terms, produce justice of any kind for the white working class, or the most deprived among the white working class? These are substantive questions that will require more detailed treatment in subsequent chapters but they are raised here to highlight some of the difficulties that attach to inter-group comparisons and the assessment of justice between groups.[14]

THE CHARACTERISTICS OF AFFIRMATIVE ACTION

A characterisation of affirmative action can be arrived at by the following steps – which are a summary of what has gone before. The starting point is the perceived under-representation or under-utilisation of the affected groups in desired positions and statuses. This, it is argued, has arisen in large measure as a result of the inequality of opportunity that these groups have enjoyed (and continue to enjoy) and this in turn is a consequence of negative discrimination, both direct and indirect, intentional and unintentional, and of relative disadvantage manifested in greater or different needs from those of the majority group (or groups). Logic then dictates that a remedial strategy must be targeted at the affected groups or at practices which discriminate against the groups. It must be groups and not individuals that will benefit. The affected groups are potentially many in number but, with the exception of the disabled, all will be defined or identified by criteria which are morally arbitrary. It is this factor – the moral arbitrariness of the beneficiary groups – that makes such remedial practices (which we have called race-conscious practices) prima facie unjust. However, insofar as remedial practices are directed at meeting needs (to reduce disadvantage) it may be argued that the greater or special needs of these groups justifies their selection for benefit and that the morally arbitrary criterion by which members are identified is really just a proxy for the morally relevant criterion of need. This formulation however makes the 'justification' of a morally arbitrary criterion contingent upon empirical circumstances (and ones that will always be contestable). Morally speaking, therefore, race-conscious practices must remain at least prima facie unjust ones and this remains their distinguishing feature in the domain of public policy and what sets them aside from 'ordinary good practice'.

The final step in this conceptual derivation of affirmative action requires that it be detached, so far as is possible, from cognate practices such as preferential treatment. Both practices share the prima-facie unjustness of aiming to benefit morally arbitrary groups. This factor alone will not set one apart from the other. Where a difference may be found is in the procedures each practice adopts to achieve its ends. Procedures that override the requirements of 'justice' in respect either of the merit principle or of the needs principle we would call preferential treatment. Such practices would include hiring or promoting less well qualified minority group members over better qualified majority group members, or allocating resources to minority groups in a volume that takes them beyond equality of welfare at the expense of meeting the needs of the majority group (or some of its members). A crucial qualification to this formulation however is that 'merit' is a very dubious contender as a material principle of justice. To override merit may well be unfair, but it is doubtful that it can be called unjust.

What characterises affirmative action procedures is that, unlike preferential treatment, they do not override the demands of 'justice' or fairness in respect either of merit or needs principles. Affirmative action therefore identifies beneficiary groups (or members of groups) by morally arbitrary criteria but thereafter, in theory at least, everything it does lies within the boundaries of justice or fairness. In practice, as we have noted, a large grey area exists at the boundary of affirmative action and preferential treatment.

3 The logic of affirmative action

As a prerequisite of any evaluation of affirmative action it will be necessary to make more explicit what it is intended to achieve (and whether these goals are realistic both in theory and in practice), the logic which connects affirmative action practice to these goals, the means and methods that it uses, and the constraints which may limit its effective reach. Each of these will be treated in turn, but for present purposes it will be sufficient only to draw attention to the potential limitations of affirmative action because these will be the subject of more extensive treatment in later chapters.

At one level, a superficial one, the purposes and procedures of affirmative action are clear enough. We can derive from the previous chapter the simple formula that affirmative action is used in circumstances of demonstrated minority under-representation in order to reduce that under-representation by means of outreach, encouragement, training and so on. But this superficial rendering is inadequate for a number of reasons, not the least of which is a lack of any precision about the goals to be achieved and how progress towards them is to be measured or about how the procedures of affirmative action will operate in practice to reach the desired ends. On closer inspection, these turn out to be far from obvious. The simple formulation of the logic of affirmative action also fails to take account of the vexatious question of who the beneficiaries are and who they should be. Is it enough, for example (with current practice, it has to be), that *any* members of minority groups should benefit so long as minority representation is increased, or does justice (or 'fair play') require that the members of minority groups who benefit be those in greatest need, or suffering the worst disadvantage or who have been harmed most by past discrimination? I have rehearsed these arguments elsewhere in respect of positive discrimination (Edwards 1987); they will need to be resurrected in the context of affirmative action programmes.

THE GOALS OF AFFIRMATIVE ACTION

There are two quite different types of goal that have been customarily attached to the practices of affirmative action and preferential treatment, and a number of others that we shall want to add. We shall first consider the two more customary goals. These have been characterised as forward- and backward-looking goals (Goldman 1976), the former focusing on the promotion of equality of opportunity by relief from discrimination and the meeting of needs, whilst the latter emphasises the remedial nature of the practices as means of compensating for past harm and injustice resulting from negative discrimination. The two types of practice are not equally suited to the achievement of both goals however; affirmative action is, in most circumstances, more appropriate for enhancing equality of opportunity, whilst preferential treatment (which anyway will often override the formal requirements of equality of opportunity) will be more effective in bringing about compensation. That having been said, both practices can be, and are, used in pursuit of both goals, though, as we shall see, compensatory arguments are less common (and less popular) than arguments for greater equality of opportunity.

To characterise the goals of affirmative action in this way, however, is to lend it an aura of moral respectability that it does not always possess. Both of the goals we have cited may be seen in their own way to be fulfilling the requirements of justice – meeting needs for its own sake or in pursuit of greater equality of opportunity, and acknowledging rights to compensation for past harm. Both of these, as we have seen, are material principles of formal distributive justice. But these are the articulated, manifest aims of affirmative action. There are other (often but not always) latent goals which, on the occasions when they do appear in the rhetoric of affirmative action, seem to have been introduced to appeal to particular constituencies for whom calls to justice would cut little ice. This seems particularly to be the case when affirmative action is seen as an instrument for achieving greater equality of opportunity and perhaps for this reason appeals to consequence rather than justice are more common in the language of affirmative action in Great Britain than in America. If, therefore, we tie affirmative action closely to the pursuit of equality of opportunity (as we must), then we must also attach to it the reasons and purposes of seeking greater equality of opportunity – which will not always be justice-regarding. And for this reason, we shall have to subdivide the goal of equality of opportunity into its deontic and consequential sub-components. Thus, for example, the Commission for Racial Equality lists the following benefits for industry from an equal opportunity policy (which, if properly implemented, would include affirmative action practices): better staff, better communications within the organisation, better industrial relations, better employee relations, 'better image in the community', better use of staff, better business and better service, and 'more efficient procedures' (Commission for Racial Equality 1989: 32–35). The Institute of Personnel Management notes (as we might expect) that

> The regrettable results [of continuing discrimination] are increasingly apparent in disillusionment among ethnic minorities and women, in social unrest and, most important in the employment context, *in the misuse and/or waste of human resources.*
>
> (Institute of Personnel Management 1986, emphasis original)

We can recognise in these encomiums the appeals to self-interest that are required to sell equal opportunity policies to less than enthusiastic buyers.

We need not dwell at this point on the consequential components of affirmative action; there is more to be said about the two apodictic aims that we have identified, and in particular about the differing emphasis given to them in the two countries under consideration. Much of the philosophical debate in the USA about both practices revolved, at least until about ten years ago, around the question of compensation (see for example Bayles 1973b, Fullinwider 1980, Goldman 1979, Blackstone 1977). And even though both Title VII of the Civil Rights Act 1964 and Executive Order 11246 are silent on the matter, courts have used the former to impose specifically remedial quotas (even though they go under the name of goals) for egregious past discrimination, or to give legal blessing to consent decrees for the same purpose, as in *United States v. Paradise* (1987) and *Local 93 of the International Association of Firefighters v. City of Cleveland* (1986), the latter of which also gave support to the permissibility of benefiting minority group members who were not themselves the victims of discriminatory injustice.

The compensation issue receives less of an airing in the US today than in the past, but that does not mean that it is moribund. In Great Britain by contrast, apart from the occasional rhetorical utterance, the question of taking remedial action to compensate groups for past harm has hardly surfaced. The Race Relations Act 1976 of course makes provision for legal compensation for *individual* acts of discrimination but compensation as a *group* practice is not entertained despite the occasional reference to it as in the influential Plowden Report (Plowden 1967: 57) where it is used to mean 'making up for past disadvantage' rather than as remedy or reparation, or in the assertion by the CRE (1985a:36) that 'Positive action should be a remedy for past disadvantage that is a complement to, rather than a substitute for, a general programme for ending discrimination', which, again, should be read as making up for disadvantage rather than compensating for the harm caused by discrimination.

Again, we shall leave aside any substantive discussion of whether remedial compensation *is* owed to ethnic minority groups in Great Britain and simply note that the idea of remedial compensation is not in fact entertained there either legislatively or politically.

However, we cannot so easily escape from the dilemma about the purposes of positive action that results from the tension between compensation on the one hand and promoting equality of opportunity on the other. If compensation for harm resulting from past (and present) discrimination is not acceptable as a reason for promoting affirmative action, we are still left with the problem of what exactly causes the disadvantage, the removal of which, in pursuit of equality of opportunity, now remains the only (or the main) justification. There was a time when the 'newness' argument about recent immigrant arrivals could be evidenced, but this is no longer tenable. And even when we have taken account of all the other possible explanations outlined in Chapter 2, there remain the effects of discrimination. It just is not feasible to account for the relative disadvantage of ethnic minorities without some recourse to negative discrimination as one causal factor. We must then ask, should the costs and the benefits of this discrimination be allowed to lie where they fall other than to the extent of the quixotic ameliorations of need-based positive action? Should nothing be done to satisfy the demands of justice that harm be remedied and that rights overridden be recompensed, other than to ameliorate some of the disadvantage that is a consequence?[1] The formal answer to these questions would be that of course hurt should be compensated, as indeed it is under the Race Relations Act in Great Britain and Title VII and the Fourteenth Amendment in the USA. But these (and the former in particular) place a heavy emphasis on direct and intentional discrimination and rather less on indirect discrimination (see Lustgarten and Edwards 1992). So far as the law is concerned (as must be the case) there need to be identifiable victims and perpetrators to whom can be attached intent or, at least, culpability. This severely limits both in principle and in practice the amount of hurt that can be compensated. And this is further compounded in Great Britain by the absence of class actions, which, in the USA, have the effect of ringing the tocsin for discriminating agencies. But even if all identifiable cases of discrimination could be rectified by the law – either in courts or tribunals – the assumption underlying legal action is a partial one; it is an assumption that discrimination (direct and indirect) consists of a number of discrete acts of malfeasance, whether intentional or not. There is an alternative (or supplementary) view of discrimination that sees it as endemic in society, as part of a deeply rooted racism, and as institutional rather than aberrational (see for example McCrudden, Smith and Brown 1991, Ball and Solomos 1990, Braham, Rattansi and Skellington 1992, Rex 1988). On this view, discrimination and the harm it causes are far too widespread and endemic to be susceptible to the reach of law, given its insistence upon discrete acts. If this is the case then a great deal (possibly a very great deal) of discrimination and injury goes uncompensated for.

The question therefore remains – must the costs and the benefits of this discrimination be allowed to lie where they fall? Despite the perceived public and political unacceptability of a compensatory function for affirmative action, is it possible that it *could* achieve this end? Could compensation be one of the goals of affirmative action? Perhaps one of the strongest arguments against affirmative action (and preferential treatment) as a compensatory mechanism that has been voiced in the USA is that it is a very inefficient way of achieving justice – and a poor approximation to justice at that. It is a group practice, but one that, in the employment field at least, does not benefit the whole group but only those members, quixotically selected (in terms of justice), who are in a position to take advantage of the affirmative or preferential measures taken. There is no reason to believe that those who benefit most are the ones who would do so under a pure system of compensation, or who are the most deserving of compensation, and some reason to believe that there is an approximate inverse relation between desert for and receipt of compensation. Conversely, those who pay the costs of affirmative action or preferential treatment – whites who do not get jobs that they otherwise would or who are made redundant when seniority rules are overridden to preserve minority affirmative action gains – are not necessarily those most guilty of negative discrimination against minorities (see Lynch 1989, Carter 1991, Sowell 1990, Simon 1977, Goldman 1979, Greene 1977, Gross 1977, Hoffman 1977). Now, so far as I am aware, that these assertions are empirically supportable has never been challenged, but they have led to a debate (which we shall not enter here) about whether it is not anyway the whole of a minority group or groups who have been discriminated against and harmed, and all whites (some say white men) who are guilty of the discrimination. Compensation is therefore owed to all Afro-Americans, Hispanics, American Indians, etc. and the costs ought to be borne by all whites (or all white males).

The logic of this position then permits the argument that since we are dealing with whole-group harm and the need for whole-group compensation, a *group* practice such as affirmative action or preferential treatment is almost tailor-made to bring about a better balance of justice. That these practices are indifferent to the distribution of benefits and costs *within* groups does not (on this argument) compromise justice. Furthermore, because discrimination is endemic and institutionalised, it is impossible anyway to identify individual victims, and even less so individual culprits. Group practices therefore are not only appropriate compensatory mechanisms, they are the *only* ones.

There are several difficulties with these arguments (which have only been presented in very summary form here), not least of which is a specification of harmed and harming groups and the relatively indiscriminate manner in which the 'oppressed' and the oppressors are identified (are white women, for example, innocent of discrimination against ethnic minorities?). Our present purpose, however, is to establish whether compensation should or could be one of the goals of affirmative action practice and it is my belief that the strengths of the arguments outlined above are such at least as to establish a prima-facie case that affirmative action (and perhaps even more so, preferential treatment) type practices *could* be used as compensatory mechanisms. Whether they *should* must remain subject to a weighing up of the demands of justice, but it is worth noting in this respect that the principal charge against affirmative action as compensation – that it is indifferent to the distribution of remedies and costs within groups – is one that could equally well be levelled against the practice when used for 'acceptable' reasons – the promotion of equality of opportunity. It is as indifferent to degrees of need (and who possesses them) as it is to degrees of desert for compensation (and who possesses them).

The aversion to using affirmative action for compensatory purposes that is evident in both Great Britain and (to a lesser extent) America would not appear, therefore, to be based on any considered view about its capacity to achieve this end. There are flaws in the argument for group compensation but they are not, on first view at least, fatal.

Thus far, we have concentrated on compensation and equality of opportunity as goals of affirmative action, the latter of which we have subdivided into its deontic and consequential components. There are three other identifiable goals that any near-rigorous evaluation of affirmative action must acknowledge. These are the promotion of diversity, enhancing the general status and quality of life of minorities, and advancing distributive justice. The latter two are so closely related, however, that they can, for the purposes of evaluation, be combined.

'Diversity' has come to refer to the end result of a process of increasing the range and variability of personnel in organisations, companies, institutions and occupations. It has found more resonance in the United States (where it first surfaced somewhat under a decade ago) than in Great Britain, though the kindred, but not identical, notion of multiculturalism has gained some standing in Great Britain (see Commission for Racial Equality 1982, Burney 1988, Swann 1985).

'Encouraging diversity' brings a more abstract (if not ethereal) dimension to the goals of affirmative action. It refers only superficially to numerical diversity of employees or faculty or students and more fundamentally to such notions as a 'rich diversity of cultures' and a 'diversity of perspectives and approaches'. And like equality of opportunity, it is sometimes promoted as an end (and a good) in itself and sometimes as a means to other ends (cultural enrichment, better decision-making, greater productivity and so on). We must bear in mind, therefore, that diversity may be subdivided into its deontic and consequential components.

The diversity of 'Diversity' in the US varies considerably from one institution to another with universities tending to be more inclusive than public sector agencies which in turn will tend to adopt a wider remit than private sector agencies. As a minimum, however, cultural diversity will include women and ethnic minorities, and the more inclusive lists will add sexual orientation (specifically homosexuals and bisexuals), the disabled, the elderly and veterans. However, what is not made clear in documents extolling the virtues of diversity – and what is of importance to the current task of articulating the goals of affirmative action – is whether the demands of diversity are the same as the demands of compensation or of equality of opportunity in terms of *which* groups should be included. Given that the rationale for diversity is the 'cultural enrichment' of an organisation that flows from the presence in it of a multitude of 'human groups', it does not necessarily seem to be the case that the variety of these groups should be confined to the previously or currently under-represented. It may be argued, of course, that the remainder of the diversity of groups available to an organisation (that is, those *not* under-represented) need not be targeted by affirmative action just because they *are* already represented. But that may well be a specious argument. There will, in respect of many, and possibly most, organisations, be a variety of groups who are under-represented but are not included in what are called the 'affected' groups. Should we, therefore, in pursuit of diversity, try to attract to organisations more Jewish people; or Poles or Italians, or Germans, or Scandinavians, or Catholics, or Protestants, Baptists, Anabaptists, Mormons and so on? Is not the cultural tradition that Scandinavians or Catholics can bring to diversity as enriching as that of homosexuals?

The other goal at which affirmative action might be aimed is a more general one. We might see the practice as one means of effecting some redistribution of resources to minority groups in order to improve their general standing in society and their quality of life and, in the process, of enhancing distributive justice. (Such redistribution would also of course be a means to other ends – such as promoting equality of opportunity or creating role models (see Commission for Racial Equality 1985b, Exum 1983).) In reality this tends to be a portmanteau goal and one we may use for convenience when affirmative action is called in aid of the promotion of greater 'racial equality'.

Used in this way, affirmative action is more likely to involve the targeting of resources on minority groups (or on areas in which they are concentrated) rather than the sorts of procedures it uses to promote equality of opportunity or diversity or to compensate. And to the extent that this is the case, it must rest upon certain assumptions about the nature, discreteness and relative quantity of minority needs compared with the majority population. These are questions that we have tried to answer in the previous chapter and they need not be aired again here.

SOME FURTHER ENDS

A part of the evaluation of affirmative action must involve a clarification of how it works and this in turn requires a better specification of means and ends. Thus far, we have identified five broad aims for affirmative action: compensation, equality of opportunity as an end in itself and as a means to other ends, diversity, and racial equality or justice. These do not all function as 'ultimate goals', however, and equality of opportunity in particular, though some sort of 'good' in itself, is ultimately a means of increasing the representation of minority group members in institutions and occupations. It would seem – at least on a first analysis – that we use affirmative action to promote equality of opportunity in order to increase representation *and* in order to compensate *and* to promote diversity. Equality of opportunity, it would appear, is as much a means to other ends as an end in itself. It is also used (though using different affirmative action procedures) to help promote ethnic minority businesses, which may also be viewed as an end in itself or a means of improving the social and economic status of minorities or of producing role models. The function that the promotion of equality of opportunity plays in this is the removal of barriers to access to capital for setting up businesses, the use of set-asides, provision of advice and so on (Commission for Racial Equality 1981a: 9, Greater London Enterprise Board 1985: 6).

We find, therefore, when we try to pin down the goals that we hope to achieve with affirmative action, a complex interplay of ends and means and the risk of ever-receding 'ultimate' goals. (We shall also find that the goal of 'greater minority representation' (for which the promotion of equality of opportunity is a means) is itself problematical.) As a first stage in clarifying these relationships therefore, and of making the 'logic of affirmative action' more explicit, the interrelationship between the various means and goals are represented in Figure 3.1.

Like all diagrammatic representations this is an over-simplification of what is in effect a fluid and complex set of relationships. We use affirmative action procedures (of which more later) in order to promote equality of opportunity or to meet needs (either as an end or as one means of creating more equality of opportunity). Greater equality of opportunity, it is assumed, will, among many other things, increase minority group representation, promote minority businesses and act as compensation. (This last however may be more directly accomplished

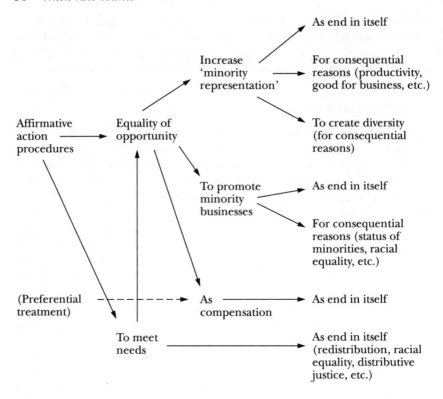

Figure 3.1 Affirmative action: means and goals

by means of preferential treatment which will by-pass the equal opportunity stage.)

Increased minority representation,[2] so the logic goes, may represent
an end in itself or, as we have noted, it may be pursued for other and
further reasons such as increased productivity, better workforce relations
and so on, or third, as a means of creating more diversity in workforces,
faculties or student bodies, which may itself be a means to other ends.

The encouragement of more minority businesses may in turn be seen
either as an end in itself (as self-evidently 'good') or once more as a
means to other ends such as improving the status and quality of life of
minority group members or promoting 'racial equality'.

Where equality of opportunity is seen as a means of compensation
for past harm it will normally best be seen as an end in itself, fulfilling
a requirement of justice, and not as a means to other ends.

Finally, when affirmative action is used to meet needs, it may be seen
as contributing to greater equality of opportunity (as, for example,
through skills training) or, again, as an end in itself by way of fulfilling
the needs principle of justice and hence promoting racial equality or
distributive justice.

MINORITY REPRESENTATION

Thus far, 'under-representation' has been used as a shorthand to include a number of different ends (or more precisely, measures of 'success'). These need now to be disaggregated because they differ not only as numerical measures but also in the assumptions about the nature of equality of opportunity upon which they are based. The most important distinction, however, and the one on which we shall concentrate, is that between 'under-representation' and 'under-utilisation'. These differ not only as measures of relative minority presence in occupations and positions, but more fundamentally in the (often implicit) assumptions they use about what the appropriate presence should be. Under-utilisation is also a more precise concept than under-representation. The difficulty with the latter is that it is often used imprecisely and with a variety of correlates. If we wish to increase the proportion of minority group members in an institution or occupation (say a large company), we must first have evidence of the degree of under-representation or utilisation and some idea of what the 'appropriate' representation would be in the absence of all those factors which we believe have compromised fair equality of opportunity. A rough approximation of the expected representation in a workforce would take account of representation in the labour draw area, age structures, required qualifications and so on. We find in practice, however, representations expressed with no apparent logic or consistency in relation to the minority population as a whole, in a particular locality, in the workforce, in the travel to work area and so on. There is no consensus on how representation ought to be calculated.

Clearly, what is at issue therefore with representativeness is what the proportion of minorities should be *representative of*, and this is both an empirical and a conceptual matter. Empirically, it makes all the difference if what one is aiming to achieve is a minority presence that reflects their representation in the population as a whole or in the working population or in the labour force or in the labour catchment area of a particular plant. The appropriate targets for minority representation will vary in each case – and, depending on the measure, vary drastically. A representation that reflects minority presence in the population as a whole might be better suited when looking at a whole profession or occupation but even that will be only a very crude measure unless account is taken of the age imbalance between majority and minority groups. It would be a wholly inappropriate comparison for representation in a particular plant, particularly if it were located in an area of very high or low minority population. Comparison with minority representation in the labour force as a whole, or within a city, will in most cases be a more realistic one to make than with overall representation in the population (if only because it will take account of age imbalances) but it will still provide an inadequate and misleading indicator of what representation might reasonably be expected at a particular plant or office location. For this sort of comparison a minority presence that reflected representation in the travel-to-work area of the plant or better still representation in the labour force within the travel-to-work area would in most instances be more appropriate. But even then we may be ignoring factors (such as age distribution) which will affect representation at different points in an occupational hierarchy, educational qualifications, level of training and so forth. The more of such factors we add in, the nearer we move to the alternative measure of utilisation.

Utilisation as a measure of minority presence in institutions or organisations is best exemplified by the under-utilisation analysis required to be carried out by federal contractors in the United States as part of their Affirmative Action Plan as laid down in Executive Order 11246. Used in this context, utilisation analysis is a more precise measure than any of the variations of representation mentioned above – though it incorporates aspects of them. Essentially, the utilisation analysis compares current minority presence in a company or institution with what it could be, given equality of opportunity *under existing conditions*. It involves an analysis of eight factors relating to the labour force draw area:

• the minority population,
• minority unemployment,
• percentage of minorities in the local workforce,
• minorities with requisite job skills,
• minorities which can be recruited,
• the availability of training facilities,
• promotable or transferable persons within the employer's workforce,
• expansion, contraction and turnover in the workforce.[3]

(United States Code of Federal Regulations 1989: Title 41, Chapter 60–2.11(b) (1) (i)–(viii))

Utilisation analysis, therefore, as the name implies, provides a measure of the extent to which the existing 'utilisable' minority labour force is being employed by the contractor. The eight-factor analysis is so designed as to prevent employers being able to hide behind untested assertions that low minority representation is the result of their unavailability. It also constitutes a baseline of variables that employers must consider in order to be certain that minority representation is as high as it can be (or could be, given proper training facilities), short of trying to assess consistent differences in unconstrained job and career preferences and choices between different groups.

Under-*representation*, therefore, comes in a variety of forms but in most of these it differs from under-utilisation not only in its constituent measures but also, and more importantly, in its underlying conception of equality of opportunity. Under-utilisation operates with a much more limiting conception of equality of opportunity, based as it is on the *current availability* of minorities (but with the inclusion of potential availability resulting from training). It takes as a 'given', therefore, a current availability that will itself be the result of generations of discrimination and disadvantage, rather than attempting to assess (by counter-factual reasoning or simple proportionality) what the level of availability *would now be if past harm and disadvantage had not occurred*. Measures of under-representation on the other hand are more likely (by accident rather than design) to acknowledge a broader conception of equality of opportunity which assumes that the presence of minorities ought to be greater than current availability would suggest.

THE NATURE OF AFFIRMATIVE ACTION GOALS

Clearly, the interlocking goals of affirmative action differ considerably in their moral standing (as well as in their place in the 'logic of affirmative action'). Some are means to other ends, others represent ends in themselves and yet others are pursued for contingent reasons. And some appear to be both ends in themselves and also means to achieving contingent ends. Our evaluation, therefore, requires that the moral standing of the goals of affirmative action be clarified and the present section attempts this by locating them on a 'moral map'. The purpose here is primarily to distinguish between aims and goals that are morally prescriptive in the sense that justice (or some other first-order principle) would require them, and those that are consequential in the sense that the purpose for pursuing them is not apodictic but because it is anticipated that they will bring about other ends which are deemed to be a 'good'. There will nonetheless be other goals which will not easily sit in either of these camps and which may in consequence have no particular moral standing.

Compensatory affirmative action is justice-regarding. If it is genuinely compensatory in motive (whether it is in practice will depend in large measure on whether it is seen to be group- or individual-based compensation), its purpose will be to correct ancient wrongs and its prescriptive character will derive from the rights to compensation that past wrongs bestow upon the victims. Affirmative action will be the instrument for seeing that these rights to compensation are fulfilled (see Fullinwider 1980, Kennedy 1986, O'Neil 1987, Boxhill 1977). If compensation for past discrimination is deemed to be due, therefore (a far from uncontested view), then the moral grounds for implementing affirmative action (and more questionably preferential treatment) are very strong.

The pursuit of equality of opportunity in its own right is usually treated as a morally worthwhile goal – as something that *ought* to be done (even though, for the purposes of palatability, it is sometimes garnished with contingent benefits), though it is not immediately clear from whence it derives its moral apodicity (see Edwards 1990a). Certainly there are some grounds for believing that equality of opportunity is a requirement of justice. We have already noted that need is a material principle of justice and that justice requires distribution in proportion to needs. Having needs is one component of inequality of opportunity and part at least therefore of what makes for such inequality is morally prescriptive. The conjunction may, however, be incidental and though meeting needs may help to equalise opportunity it may not be primarily for this reason that justice demands it.

Second, support for the apodicity of equality of opportunity can be found in Rawls's contract theory. Fair equality of opportunity constitutes the second part of Rawls's second principle of justice (and comes lexicographically prior to the Difference Principle) (Rawls 1972: 60–65, 83–87, 302–3). According to Rawls, therefore, 'veil of ignorance' contractors would include the promotion of fair equality of opportunity as one principle of justice. However, this lends only qualified support to the moral prescriptivity of equality of opportunity precisely because of Rawls's particular conception of it. 'Fair equality of opportunity' is not the same as equality of opportunity and whereas Rawls makes a convincing case that original-position contractors would contract to the former, it is unlikely that they would do so in respect of the latter. Conventionally, we may see equality of opportunity as free competition unhampered by morally or functionally arbitrary factors (such as discrimination) given the existing and actual distribution of talents and abilities. Each of us would then go as far as our capacities, preferences and drive would take us. And this is just *not* what Rawlsian contractors would agree to. *Fair* equality of opportunity on the other hand relies for its force on its conjunction with, and dependence on, the Difference Principle, which, Rawls argues, 'represents an agreement to regard the distribution of natural talents *as a common asset* and to share in the benefits of [this] distribution whatever it turns out to be' (Rawls 1972: 101, emphasis added).[4]

A third approach to the apodicity of equality of opportunity might be through the idea of rights. Goldman, for example, has argued in favour of 'rights to positions based on equal opportunity' on the grounds that:

> Unless we do establish such rights, equal opportunity will remain without significant practical effect. The right to compete for jobs on a fair basis means little if those successful in the competitions cannot claim the jobs as rights.

> (Goldman 1987: 95)

Though Goldman is here attempting to establish the idea of *rights to positions*, he is doing so by taking as axiomatic our right to compete fairly for them. Indeed, one might argue, with the same logic, the reverse of his case – that there can be no rights to positions (that is, you can have no right to the job for which you have been selected as the best qualified and most suitable) unless everyone has the right to compete for them on equal terms – that is, without some form of equal opportunity.

The right to equality of opportunity[5] might also be derived from the notion of having a right to equal consideration, which Dworkin has distinguished from the right to equal treatment (Dworkin 1981), and from what Walzer has called 'candidate rights' (Walzer 1983: 152–54). The one broadly derives from the other. If we have a right to equal consideration along with others, taking only relevant factors into account, then in the particular field of employment (or positions more generally) this will translate into the right of all candidates for a post to be given equal consideration (again taking only relevant factors into account).

These formulations of equality of opportunity as a rights-based enterprise appear at first sight to endow it with strong moral pre-scriptivity. Rights should not lightly be overridden. And so it might be were there an agreed and uncontentious view of what equality of opportunity is and – of greater importance – what all the 'relevant considerations' are and are not. Morally speaking, however, we cannot think of equality of opportunity in isolation from 'merit', which is in effect the collective name for 'relevant considerations'. And it is when we come to consider what constitutes 'merit' (which we shall do in Chapter 9) that doubts must inevitably creep in about whether we would wish people to have rights, the exercise of which and the enjoyment of the benefits from which rely so heavily on it.

Despite the not inconsiderable arguments that can be marshalled in favour of equal opportunity being considered a requirement of justice – something that we *ought* to do because justice demands it – very substantial doubts remain that this is in fact the case. It may be that justice demands *something* in respect of what governs our life-chances, but it is far from clear that it is equality of opportunity in its colloquial sense and use.

An alternative formulation, and one that is probably morally more accurate, is that whilst equality of opportunity and the merit system are too imperfect to bear the weight of moral prescriptivity, they do represent the 'rules of the game' as most participants would agree them (or would agree them were they purged of their obvious current imperfections). And playing by the rules of the game and accepting the outcome – whatever it might be – is 'fair play'. There is therefore – on this rendering – nothing morally absolute about equality of oppor-tunity; it is just something we should do because it is (would be) fair and everyone would have agreed to its being so. We consider the 'rules of the game' in more detail in Chapter 9.

Equality of opportunity appears also to be promoted for consequential, and perhaps utilitarian, reasons, as we have already noted. It is not easy to say how much of the consequential rhetoric that sometimes attaches to equal opportunity practice rests on a genuine belief that the alleged benefits really will accrue and how much on the need to sell the practice in constituencies where claims of justice or fairness carry little weight. It is a risky argument, and one whose vulnerability would easily be exposed were it to be shown that the anticipated benefits failed to materialise, because with such results the case for promoting equality of opportunity would evaporate. Even if we are forced to eschew the justice case for equality of opportunity and fall back on 'fairness', it would still be a stronger base than consequentialism, subject as that is to what must always be highly dubious evidence about a causal link between the promotion of equal opportunities on the one hand and higher productivity, greater efficiency, better workforce relations and such-like, on the other.

For present purposes, improving representation and utilisation may be treated together. Both are to be seen as the consequence of greater equality of opportunity, though this is of course not the only way in which they could be achieved (preferential quotas could produce the same result much more quickly). Like equality of opportunity, improved representation and utilisation can be both ends in themselves and means to subsequent ends. As ends in themselves they may simply be seen as the successful result of greater equality of opportunity and an indication that greater fairness had been achieved or the requirements of justice more fully met. No further justification would be required. That has not, however, prevented them from also being extolled for their consequential virtues, many of which are similar to those claimed for greater equality of opportunity.

One of the consequences of greater minority representation or utilisation might be (though would not necessarily be) more diversity, and this has increasingly been claimed as an important reason for pursuing affirmative action. Now although diversity is sometimes claimed to be a good in its own right (as well as creating contingent benefits), it cannot be said to constitute a moral good in any sense. There can be nothing of *moral* value in creating a workforce or student body that is diverse in its composition (as there would be for example in rectifying rights overridden or in meeting need). Diversity is 'good', we must assume, in the same way that 'socially balanced communities' or a 'sense of community' used to be thought of as 'good'. And like these other constructions, other than for the nice warm feeling that it induces, there is little about 'the good' that diversity produces that is not consequential in nature. Diversity, like community, may be a good

thing but ultimately its goodness lies in its real or imagined consequences and not in any inherent properties. Since warm feelings are
difficult to evaluate, we shall confine our attentions to the promotion
of diversity as a means of producing other contingent goods.

Like increased representation and utilisation, the promotion of
minority business enterprises is both an end in itself (a recognition of
greater equality of opportunity and of minority group success in an
'enterprise driven economy') and consequentially provides role models,
helps to reduce minority unemployment, enhances the standing of
minority groups and, hopefully, creates more wealth in the minority
community. The last of these, of course, represents the most tangible
end in itself.

The goals of affirmative action, therefore, present an odd mixture of
the morally deontic, the consequential and rule conformity. Some are
capable of being interpreted in more than one of these three ways and
their moral standing may depend as much (or more) on presentational
exigencies as on their inherent moral status. An evaluation of the moral
standing of affirmative action (and preferential treatment) will form
the basis of a later chapter.

THE LOGIC OF AFFIRMATIVE ACTION

It is clear from what has been said so far that other than as a direct way
of meeting needs when this is an end in itself, affirmative action, as a
goal-oriented strategy, operates in large measure by means of promoting equality of opportunity. The latter is an intermediate goal
(except when it increases minority representation as an end in itself)
and it is the primary instrument through which affirmative action
operates. The logic of affirmative action therefore is that its constituent
procedures act in a variety of ways to increase the opportunities that
minority group members can avail themselves of in order to increase
representation as an end in itself or to create more diversity or for a
number of other contingent reasons. In this section we focus on the
first part of this process – the nature of the barriers to equality of
opportunity and how affirmative action might operate to remove or
reduce them.

Equality of opportunity is a porous concept. In some of its formulations it is unattainable. In others it raises expectations that in practice
will only be partially fulfilled and no more is this the case than when
they are based in a mixture of ideological rhetoric and woolly thinking.
If affirmative action is to be of value, therefore, it must operate with a
sound and sensible version of equality of opportunity and one in
particular that recognises the limits of effective intervention. Our
immediate purpose, therefore, is the limited one of clarifying some of

the cross-cutting interpretations of equality of opportunity that bear upon our understanding of how it relates to affirmative action. Substantive discussion of equality of opportunity and related ideas is kept over to a later chapter.

Equality of opportunity has been variously interpreted as an equality of opportunity to do, or achieve, something (such as a personal life plan), as equality of chances to achieve something (a job or position or status) or as equality of results. The last of these can be despatched first. Inequalities (of income, wealth, etc.) are in large measure determined by the reward system. A successful equal opportunity strategy would result in a randomising of people's opportunities to be placed at any given point on the reward system. It would, in other words, randomise opportunities to be *unequal*. Equality of opportunity has nothing to do with equality of results (or, simply, equality).

Nor does equality of opportunity equate with equal chances of gaining a particular slot in the reward system. Equal chances come by the toss of a coin (Gross 1987: 124) and no amount of equal opportunity will give each one of us an equal *chance* of being a judge, surgeon, rap singer or whatever.

The third interpretation is the one we shall carry forward through subsequent chapters. Essentially, this is the enterprise of equalising *between individuals or groups*, those factors that affect or determine their opportunities to achieve some goal (job, status, etc. or personal plan). Broadly speaking, this is equality of opportunity as removing arbitrary barriers and compensating for compensatable deficiencies (Williams 1969). In normal usage we tacitly acknowledge that the promotion of equality of opportunity is limited to those factors that are removable and compensatable. When equality of opportunity is focused on groups rather than individuals, this constraint is sometimes lost sight of.

It is convenient to think of the pursuit of equality of opportunity in the above form, as progressing through three stages. The first is the removal of morally arbitrary barriers such as first-order sex or race discrimination. The second is to compensate for the effects of deprivation, poverty, incomplete families and so on (see Plowden Report 1967, Marris and Rein 1967, Moynihan 1969, Fishkin 1987). The third stage is the much more difficult and contentious one of compensating for genetic endowment (see Rosenberg 1987, Steiner 1987).

These distinctions are not central to the arguments in subsequent chapters but they are important ones to bear in mind, if only to avoid confusions. And this is particularly so when we come to consider the types of equal opportunity strategy (and hence affirmative action) that are appropriate for *group* as opposed to *individual* equality of opportunity.

AFFIRMATIVE ACTION AND THE CONSTRAINTS ON EQUALITY OF OPPORTUNITY

Affirmative action, therefore, operates mainly but not wholly through equality of opportunity by removing barriers to opportunity or by meeting needs so as better to enable people to compete effectively or fulfil their plans and ambitions. These represent two of the three stages in the promotion of equality of opportunity that we have identified. Affirmative action does not compensate for genetic endowments. Taking together both barriers to be removed and needs to be met along with some other factors that do not easily fit into either category, there are a large number of potential constraints that produce less than equality of opportunities and it will be necessary to familiarise ourselves with some of these before we can enter a more detailed analysis of how affirmative action is intended to work.

It will be useful to begin with a rough-and-ready classification of types of constraint:

- direct discrimination,
- indirect discrimination,
- social needs that arise from discrimination,
- special social needs of the group,
- general social needs held disproportionately by the group,
- custom,
- culture,
- tradition,
- location,
- contacts,
- geographic mobility,
- differential group abilities or talents.

Some of these have already been discussed and not all are mutually exclusive (contacts, for example, will feature as an item of indirect discrimination). We shall, therefore, concentrate in this section on what is probably the most common and most damaging constraint to equal opportunity – indirect discrimination. It is also the focus for much affirmative action practice.

Indirect discrimination is legislated against in Great Britain under the 1976 Race Relations Act. In America, Title VII of the Civil Rights Act makes no explicit reference to it though it has been recognised as a signal feature of employment litigation ever since *Griggs v. Duke Power* in 1971 under the name of 'disparate impact' or 'adverse effect'.

In Great Britain, Section 1 (1)(b) of the Race Relations Act 1976 defines indirect discrimination thus:

A person discriminates against another in any circumstances relevant for the purposes of any provision of this Act if he applies to that other a requirement or condition which he applies or would apply equally to persons not of the same racial group as that other but:

(i) which is such that the proportion of persons of the same racial group as that other who can comply with it is considerably smaller than the proportion of persons not of that racial group who can comply with it; and

(ii) which he cannot show to be justifiable irrespective of the colour, race, nationality or ethnic or national origins of the person to whom it is applied; and

(iii) which is to the detriment of that other because he cannot comply with it.

(Race Relations Act 1976: s. 1(1)(b))[6]

Though the Civil Rights Act 1964 is silent on the question of indirect discrimination, six years after Title VII of the Act came into effect (2 July 1965), the Supreme Court entered a decision in the Griggs case that effectively wrote indirect discrimination into Title VII. *Griggs v. Duke Power Co.* (1971) was the first major employment discrimination decision by the Supreme Court and revolved around whether tests and qualification requirements for progression within the company which were passed or obtained differentially between white and black groups were discriminatory. (By 1970 Duke Power had ceased to operate directly discriminatory practices.) The court's decision was unanimous and its opinion (drafted by Chief Justice Burger) on the meaning and intent of Title VII was as follows:

The objective of Congress in the enactment of Title VII is plain from the language of the statute. It was to achieve equality of employment opportunities and remove barriers that have operated in the past to favour an identifiable group of white employees over other employees. Under the Act, practices, procedures, or tests neutral on their face, and even neutral in terms of intent, cannot be maintained if they operate to 'freeze' the status quo of prior discriminatory employment practices.

(*Griggs v. Duke Power* 1971: 401 US at 429–30)

Further to emphasise the point, the opinion noted that:

The Act proscribes not only overt discrimination but also practices that are fair in form, but discriminatory in operation. *The touchstone is business necessity.* If an employment practice which operates to exclude [blacks] cannot be shown to be related to job performance, the practice is prohibited.

(*Griggs v. Duke Power* 1971: 401 US at 431, emphasis added)

In short, therefore, according to the 'Griggs doctrine', if a facially neutral practice affects different groups differently (and detrimentally to one group) and is not a practice that is *necessary* for the operation of an enterprise, it is (indirectly) discriminatory.

Much, however, hangs on the requirements of 'necessity', or 'business necessity' as it is more usually known. This will be the subject of more detailed discussion in a subsequent chapter, but it must be noted in the context of the present discussion that whilst the Commission for Racial Equality in Britain has been pressing for amendments to the Race Relations Act 1976 to incorporate a requirement of 'necessity' to replace the existing (and loose) formulation of 'justifiable' (s. 1(1)(b)(ii)) (which, as the Commission points out, has been taken by employment tribunals to include such as the costs of implementing fair practice – see Commission for Racial Equality 1985a: 2.4.1),[7] in America, the Supreme Court in *Ward's Cove Packing Co. v. Atonio* (1989) retreated from the business necessity standard to the much looser one of 'legitimate business consideration' (St Antoine 1989), and it took a new civil rights act (Civil Rights Act 1991) to reinstate the tighter formulation.

THE NATURE OF INDIRECT DISCRIMINATION

Any practice that affects one group detrimentally more than another, even if apparently neutral (in practice and intent), is indirectly discriminatory. Such a practice may however be 'justified' or 'acceptable' if it is necessary for the purposes of an enterprise (including the safety of employees and others) or, for the brief period between 1989 and 1991 in the United States, if it constituted a 'legitimate business consideration'. However, notwithstanding our earlier observation that indirect discrimination is the most damaging type of barrier to equality of opportunity, it is necessary to enter some reservations about some of the practices that have been found to be indirectly discriminatory. Given some of the profound differences between racial and ethnic groups (which in other contexts we celebrate as 'diversity'), we should not be surprised to find that there are relatively few practices which are entirely indiscriminate in their effects on different groups. And it may be (probably is) the case that in dispensing with practices that appear to discriminate between *some* groups, we have thrown out others that discriminate between groups that we might want to differentiate. Tailoring employment practices to racial neutrality both ignores the manifest differences between groups and imposes costs and limitations on our diagnostic capabilities by denying us the ability to discriminate in valuable and useful ways. That may seem a harsh (and yes, to some, racist) judgement to make so early in an evaluation of affirmative action, but evaluation is not best served by a slavish acceptance of all the assumptions upon which the practices and policies under scrutiny are based. I shall attempt in subsequent chapters to give more substance to the assertion.

For the moment, however, it is necessary to flesh out the concept of indirect discrimination with some examples. They are legion and we shall be selective. But first, one of the most bizarre examples. In 1979, in *New York City Transit Authority v. Beazer* (1979), the Supreme Court upheld the policy of the Transit Authority of not employing anyone who was a current methadone user (part of the treatment for withdrawal from heroin use). The policy had been challenged as having a discriminatory effect on blacks and Hispanics. Hence the salience of the 'business necessity' question. The vast majority of potentially or actually discriminatory practices, of course, are not as esoteric as this; they are everyday, common practices and all the more insidious for that. The most commonly cited are word-of-mouth recruiting, the use of subjective criteria and judgements at interviewing and the use of personal contacts and informal channels for recruitment (see Commission for Racial Equality 1981b, 1984, 1985c, 1989, *Equal Opportunities Review* 1985a, 1987, House of Commons 1987a, 1987b, King's Fund 1987, Wrench 1986, Levin-Epstein 1987, BACIE 1987). To these could be added the use of age requirements which will have a differential impact because of the differing age structures of minority and majority groups and, in the case of apprenticeships, because of the tendency of children from some minority groups to stay on at school beyond the maximum qualifying age; the use of restrictive catchment areas which may exclude areas of relative concentration of minorities; restricting job advertisements to sources that are less likely to be seen by minorities; the use of 'standing lists' which are activated when vacancies arise; height requirements, and so on. Other examples from the United States include a request for a photograph from job applicants, consideration of arrest records, credit status and criminal records, which have all been found to be discriminatory in circumstances where 'business necessity' could not convincingly be pleaded (see Levin-Epstein 1987).

Notwithstanding that the most pervasive forms of indirect discrimination are widespread, informal and subjective recruitment practices, it is in the area of applicant testing and qualifications that the most concerted anti-discriminatory efforts have been directed. And it is in this area, as we have seen, that concern about indirect discrimination began with the Griggs case in 1971. We shall consider the nature and impact of testing in more detail subsequently, but it is necessary here to separate out the overlapping components involved in the potentially discriminatory nature of applicant testing. There are three such components relevant to our present discussion. The first concerns tests that are not 'neutral' as between different groups – that is, people from different minority (and majority) groups pass the tests or achieve a given score at different rates. For practical purposes and for use in enforcement proceedings in the United States, the *Uniform Guidelines on Employment Selection Procedures (Uniform Guidelines* 1974) adopt what has become known as the 'four-fifths' rule and this has also been informally adopted by the Commission for Racial Equality in Great Britain (see Commission for Racial Equality 1984: 11–12). By this standard, a test is deemed to be discriminatory if the 'pass' rate, or rate of scoring at any particular mark, for a minority group is less than four-fifths of the rate for the group with the highest rate. The *Uniform Guidelines* do not say so but it has to be assumed that the group with the highest pass rate is a group identified on the same criteria as the group upon which adverse impact is being tested (race, ethnicity, sex, etc.). If then, for example, blacks perform less well as a group, on a given test, and if that test is used for job recruitment purposes, then they will be adversely affected in their likelihood of obtaining the relevant jobs.

If an employer in America is found to be using a test with adverse impact according to the four-fifths rule, then he or she must take steps (if they are federal contractors) either to use another test or adjust the offending one until neutrality is achieved, or the test must be 'validated' – that is, shown to be job-related (and hence necessary for recruitment) and not capable of substitution by another, more neutral, job-related test. There are of course problems associated with validation and neutralising tests which we have hinted at before and will further detail subsequently. The two most telling are that it has proved to be virtually impossible to devise any tests that are entirely neutral across all groups (see Blits and Gottfredson 1990a, 1990b), and that neutralising tests normally reduces their predictive capacities (see Sher 1987).

The second component concerns 'genuine occupational qualifications' (see Commission for Racial Equality 1984). By this standard, an employer should use only tests that measure capacities or abilities that are genuinely relevant to task performance in the job in question. Any other test or qualification requirement that is not directly necessary (even though it may be useful) for the performance of the job should not be used or be a requirement. In Great Britain, the 'genuine occupational qualification' issue has most often surfaced in respect of requirements about English language ability which, of course, will have an adverse affect on Asian groups.[8] What this issue raises of course is how tightly defined a genuine occupational qualification ought to be and whether it is legitimate for an employer to seek in potential employees certain qualities or abilities which, though not necessary for the performance of a job, may be beneficial to the enterprise.

The same reservation applies with even greater force to the third component of tests and qualifications. This is that it is more likely to be discriminatory of an employer if he requires of potential employees that they possess qualifications higher (or will pass tests at a higher level) than are necessary for performance of the job. We shall call this the 'maximum qualification requirement'. The discriminatory impact that it seeks to ameliorate is based on the fact (truer in America than Britain) that *some* minority groups will, on the whole, have lower levels of qualification than the majority. By requiring only the minimum qualifications necessary for the job therefore, the employer is likely to exclude from consideration fewer minority group members. Now were the maximum qualification requirement to be rigorously applied (which, on the evidence, it is not), it could have some far-reaching repercussions. Employers, for example, would not be able to take into consideration the potential promotability of applicants (something which the Supreme Court in *Griggs* left open) and universities would not be able to require more than the minimum 'A' Level grades (or less) that experience had shown were necessary for a student to pursue a degree course. Indeed, might not the maximum qualification requirement – taking not the best but the minimally qualified – be antithetical to the merit principle and the legitimate expectations that the idea of equality of opportunity has led us to believe we have? For the moment we shall reserve judgement about both whether these *are* logical (and likely) consequences of stipulating maximum qualifications, and if they are, whether they are desirable. But to tailor employment procedures to reduce their indirectly discriminatory effects is not necessarily compatible with equality of opportunity or with getting the best person for the job.

AFFIRMATIVE ACTION PRACTICES

Examples of affirmative action practice are as numerous as (and rather more numerous than) examples of indirect discrimination and other types of barrier to equality of opportunity and we should beware of including in our evaluation just anything that is done in response to an hortatory appeal to take 'affirmative' or 'positive' or 'firm' action.

In order to make our task more manageable, affirmative action procedures and practices can be classified in an approximate way as follows:

- *outreach activities*, the purpose of which is to make minority group members more aware of the possibilities open to them or to extend awareness of particular job vacancies or opportunities and which will include such measures as talks in schools or colleges with large numbers of minority students, advertising positions in the ethnic minority press, 'networking' within minority groups and so on;
- *training*, designed to qualify more minority group members for more positions (and promotions) and, like outreach, intended to

bring more qualified minorities to the interview room – this is the only form of affirmative action for which specific provision is made in the 1976 Race Relations Act under sections 35, 37 and 38, though its provision is by no means confined to designees under the Act (see Cross 1987a, 1987b);

- *neutral selection procedures* which are intended to overcome the discriminatory effects of unformalised selection processes, subjective judgements at interview, culturally biased tests and so on. This type of affirmative action will be as much concerned with devising overall neutral procedures as with identifying and stopping existing discriminatory practice;
- *goals and timetables*, which are best seen as part of the overall affirmative action process rather than as specific procedures. They provide the incentive to action and a measure of the degree of its success;
- *reducing barriers*, a wide-ranging group of activities (which also overlaps with some of the others listed here) designed to identify discriminatory selection procedures and to exhort employers to replace them with more formalised and neutral ones. Such activities will in large measure be directed at the sorts of indirectly discriminatory practices we have already identified;
- *contract compliance and grant compliance*, the legal scope for the use of which was severely curtailed under the Local Government Act 1988, provided (and to a limited extent still provides) for local authorities to require of private sector contractors or voluntary sector recipients of grant that they employ a certain proportion of minority group members in any contracted undertaking that requires the employment of new or additional personnel (see for example Burney 1988, Carr 1987, Commission for Racial Equality 1987a, 1987b, Inner London Education Authority 1986, Institute of Personnel Management 1987a, 1987b). Contract compliance is in effect a means of putting pressure on private sector employers to make special efforts to increase minority representation in their workforce, but like goals and timetables may be seen as part of an overall affirmative action practice;
- *local labour contracts* are a less controversial, legally unproblematic and altogether more anodyne way of achieving the same end as contract compliance. As the name implies, the purpose is to encourage (and, wherever possible, seek agreements with) local contractors (and even non-contractors) to employ a certain percentage of local residents on a particular project. This need not, of course, be done in pursuit of increasing minority representation (it may be a deprived area with high unemployment rates) but where there is a large minority population in the area, it may be used as a proxy for increasing their representation;
- *minority business promotion* we have already touched on. It may be achieved by advice centres for minority businesses, set-aside loans for

small business ventures and contract set-asides by local governments whereby a certain number or dollar value of contracts are given to minority businesses. Such would be of dubious legality in Britain and since *Richmond v. Croson* in 1989 has been legally more circumscribed in the United States;

- *targeted need-meeting*, which, as we have noted, must, in order to count as affirmative action, be directed solely at those needs that minority groups have as a result of the negative discrimination they have suffered or which are peculiar to the group or held in greater proportion by the group than by others and the majority group.

This is not an exhaustive classification of affirmative action – we shall come across other examples and other types in subsequent chapters – but it covers the great majority of types of practice that are common in Great Britain and the United States. It represents therefore the bulk of the armoury of affirmative action that may be brought to bear, not only (but mainly) against indirect discrimination, but also against the other limitations on equality of opportunity that we have identified in this chapter.

4 Affirmative action in employment
The British experience

In this chapter we provide some illustrative examples of affirmative action practice in both public and private sectors in the context of equal employment opportunities in Great Britain. Details of the numbers and types of organisations selected, the methods of selection and the types of data made available are included in the Appendix. Two general points need to be made here however. It was a condition of co-operation of a small number of institutions that they not be identified by name. Rather, therefore, than identify some and not others, all have been anonymised with the use of an alphabetical cipher. (The nature of the information is such, however, that the identity of some will necessarily become apparent.)

The second point is that the example institutions are not treated as self-contained case studies and are not intended to be representative. Nonetheless, it has proved to be both simpler and more productive of information to treat each institution sequentially. The main themes that derive from the treatments of institutions in both Britain and America are then summarised in Chapter 7.

THE PUBLIC SECTOR

The City of A metropolitan district

This is an authority in the north of England with a large ethnic minority population in 1991 of some 75,900 within the metropolitan district – some 16.3 per cent of the total population. The predominant groups are Asian but there is a small but significant (in race relations terms) Afro-Caribbean population.

The authority first declared itself an equal opportunities employer in 1982 in the wake of the civil unrest of 1981 and a growing concern on the part of the ruling Labour Party that insufficient attention was being paid to the needs and level of representation in the council of the large minority population. The new Race Equality and Employment policy was introduced in February 1982 and this saw the beginning of an annual headcount of minority employees of the council (City of A 1988b).[1]

Probably the most significant part of A's race and equality policy, however, in the period up to 1988 when the Conservatives gained control, was the establishment of the Race Relations Advisory Group which became very influential in policy matters and had to be consulted on all important (and in practice most less important) policy issues. This was an all-member group with only the Community Relations Council being represented from outside the authority.

In 1988, however, when the Conservatives came to power, virtually all the existing race relations apparatus was dismantled and the place allotted to race policy was very marginal. Not only was there to be a reorganisation of departments and lines of responsibility in the authority, but its style of operation was to be revolutionised. The new style was outlined in the *Strategic Plan* for 1989/90 and beyond (City of A 1989b) and the necessary structural and procedural changes, including the adoption of directorate 'Business Plans', were scheduled in a further and fuller document for the Policy and Resources Committee (City of A 1989c). Nowhere in these business plans, or anywhere else in the documents detailing the 'revolution' in the nature and style of A's procedures, was there any mention of race or equal opportunity policies. But notwithstanding its apparent disappearance, race-conscious policy did continue in A after 1988. A metropolitan district with a sixth of its population belonging to ethnic minorities, the great majority of whom belonged to non-Western cultures and whose needs were thereby at least in part distinctive, could not, whatever its political predilections, pretend that they were of no policy relevance whatsoever. And indeed, after 1988 policy changed in such a way as to put the needs of the authority's minority population (or customers as they now became) more at centre stage than had previously been the case when the focus of attention had been the ethnic make-up of the authority's own employees. This was reflected in an authority-wide race relations policy statement that emerged in 1989, the sentiments of which individual Race Relations Action Plans were to give voice to. The essential elements of this statement can be culled from two council documents of that year.

The Council's major contribution to the promotion of good race relations shall be through the provision of its essential services:

a) Council services shall be relevant to the needs of A's multicultural community;

b) the Council shall ensure equal access to those services and guarantee that no individual be disadvantaged in their receipt of services because of their cultural background;

c) the danger of creating divisions within the community through dual systems of service provision is recognised and will be avoided;

d) the right of individuals to choose their own lifestyles shall be respected. The Council recognises that the services it delivers are to meet the needs of individuals and shall not support policies which advocate the artificial preservation of cultural identities to the detriment of individual choice;

e) service provision shall be monitored to ensure the Council's policy on race relations is maintained.

The same document goes on, in a style that reflects the entrepreneurial language of the government's approach to inner-city policies (see Deakin and Edwards 1993):

Policies which further the prosperity of the District as a whole are indivisible from policies which further the prosperity of individuals within cultural minority groups. Everyone benefits by Council policies which facilitate continued economic growth, urban regeneration and housing renewal. The Council acknowledges the leading role it must play in promoting the opportunities of all in the District:

a) positive attitudes towards self-reliance and wealth creation shall be encouraged;

b) the Council shall promote equal opportunities in the District by example and shall maintain its equal opportunity employment policy;

c) the education young people receive in A will equip them with the necessary skills to take the opportunities open to them. In order that the opportunities of British society are equal, all our young people must have fluency in the English language . . .

(City of A 1989a)

We can recognise in this the ideology of entrepreneurialism that developed during the 1980s such that race relations were no longer just a matter of ensuring adequate and sensitive services, but also of ensuring opportunities for self-reliance. And one correlate of this (as with much inner-city policy) was a belief in the effectiveness of independence and self-help in promoting social change.

Race Relations Action Plans are prepared by each division within a directorate. They vary considerably in length and content (as would be expected from the new emphasis on service provision and the differential involvement of divisions in that), but most follow the same general format: a report on the monitoring of the previous twelve months' activities; an outline of new initiatives in respect of service provision for the next twelve months along with targets; and an employment position statement providing details of minority representation in the division, targets for the year and action planned to achieve these (all personnel matters having been devolved to directorates). Since our concern in this chapter is with employment practices,

we shall concentrate here on the last of these. Again, since most of the
employment components of the action plans are similar in nature
(though not, of course, quantitatively), one example will suffice to
provide the necessary 'flavour'. Having then identified a range of
affirmative action practices used in equal employment opportunity, we
will provide summary data for the authority as a whole on minority
representation.

The *Race Relations Profile and Action Plan 1989/90* (City of A 1989d)
for the Directorate of Legal Services first notes that the previous plan
set a number of targets and objectives in three areas of activity:
employment targeting, positive action initiatives and the introduction
of good personnel/managerial practice.[2] On the first of these, the plan
argues that employment targeting had proved to be effective in ensuring
that 'race equality is considered during the recruitment and selection
of prospective employees', though it does not elaborate on just what
affirmative action or other steps were taken. Targets for ethnic minority
employees in the Directorate in 1987 and 1988 had been exceeded but
in 1989 minority representation fell just short of the target. Subsequent
analysis from monitoring data indicated that the 1989 shortfall resulted
from relatively high attrition rates for minority staff (almost twice as
high as for UK white staff) and had resulted despite a continuing
increase in minority appointments both absolutely and relative to white
appointments. The Directorate's plan then attributes much of its
success in attracting minority staff to two training initiatives for young
people – the Positive Action Traineeships and the Junior Recruitment
Scheme, which between them added six minority staff to the Directorate's complement. Where most progress needs to be made, the plan
then asserts, is in getting more minority group members into senior
positions in the Directorate, where they are very few in number. Finally,
on the topic of good personnel practice, the plan notes continuing
efforts to maintain a race sensitivity in selection procedures, the
introduction of personal development training for ethnic minority
staff, and the intention of establishing a support and advice group –
again for ethnic minority staff. This review of progress is then followed
by the targets for 1989/90 which are in three parts: a proportion of
ethnic minority staff of 11 per cent (one percentage point higher than
the previous year but unrelated to any baseline data or availability
figures); a continuing review of minority employees' career progression
and assistance by means of training; and the identification of additional
areas where traineeships might be developed.

The Race Relations Profile and Action Plans of other directorates
were broadly similar to that of Legal Services and collectively they
represent potentially valuable steps to boost minority representation.
There must be some doubt, however, about the priority afforded to this
strategy. The Business Plans for the directorates, for example, are silent

on the matter of race and neither are racial matters included in directorates' performance indicators.

Affirmative action in A

The most commonly used affirmative action practices across all divisions and directorates in A in respect of employment in the authority are listed below. Most, though not all, of these are used by most divisions and directorates.

- positive action traineeships under sections 37 and 38 of the Race Relations Act 1976,
- setting employment targets and monitoring procedures,
- checking all recruitment tests and procedures to ensure that they contain no racial bias,
- provision of race awareness and sensitivity training (particularly for those involved in recruitment and selection),
- personal development training for ethnic minority employees,
- outreach work into schools, colleges, community centres, etc. to attract more ethnic minority applicants for jobs in the council,
- targeting job advertisements in the ethnic minority press and translated into minority languages.

Some directorates (and some divisions within directorates) have been more assiduous than others in the use of these affirmative action practices to increase ethnic minority representation in the council – and of course, it must be said, that it is easier for some than for others, depending on the numbers and proportions of employees in different grades (it is easier to recruit minority staff into manual and lower clerical grades than into managerial and professional posts).

How, then, has the city of A fared in its attempts to increase the proportion of its employees who come from ethnic minorities?

Ethnic minority representation in A

In the five years leading up to the 'new regime' in 1988, considerable progress had been made in the employment of ethnic minorities in most directorates, though, as Table 4.1 shows, it had been patchy. However, these proportions remain small when the (admittedly crude) comparison is made with the proportion of the metropolitan district population who were from ethnic minorities in 1987 – a figure of 21 per cent (City of A 1988a: 1). This, however, is age-unadjusted and does not give any indication of what proportion of the authority's workforce might be expected to be from ethnic minorities – except that the magnitude of the difference between an authority figure of 4.8 per cent

Table 4.1 Ethnic minority representation in A's workforce, 1982 and 1987, by directorate and whole authority

Directorate	Percentage of workforce who were Asian, Afro-Caribbean or 'other' non-UK or European	
	1982	*1987*
Legal Services[a]	0	8.2
Personnel	2.5	8.8
Finance	4.9	8.3
Housing and Env. Health	1.3	6.5
Works	0.9	2.9
Social Services	2.5	4.6
Employment and Env. Services[b]	2.2	7.3
Educational Services	2.1	4.6
Authority total	2.1	4.8

Source: City of A (1988b: 15)
Notes: (a) Legal Services was created from the City Solicitors and Chief Executive's Departments in 1987. In 1982 these two departments combined had no ethnic minority staff.
(b) Employment and Environmental Services took over from the Development Department in 1987. The 1982 figure is for the Development Department.

and the population figure of 21 per cent is such as to provide prima-facie evidence of significant under-representation.

The London Borough of B

The London Borough of B first introduced an equal opportunities policy in 1979 partly in response to pressure from minority ethnic groups in its population which in turn were using the vehicle of a highly condemnatory report on discrimination in local authority housing in the borough by the Commission for Racial Equality (London Borough of B 1990: 5). At that time 35 per cent of the borough's population were from minority ethnic groups but only 8 per cent of the council's total workforce were from these groups. Despite the fact that much of the original impetus for an equal opportunities policy came from a damaging report on service delivery (housing) however, the initial policy concentrated almost exclusively on employment within the council, and though the emphasis has shifted in recent years, this bias remains today.

An Equal Opportunities Panel was established to develop and begin to implement the policy and one of the first substantive outcomes was agreement in 1981 to set equality targets for employment within the borough council. The percentage of the council workforce who were from ethnic minorities was to double the 1981 figure of 11.5 per cent by 1983 and a minimum of 10 per cent minority representation at

Senior Officer Grade 1 level and above by December 1985. These targets were subsequently revised (in 1984) to include 35 per cent minority representation across the council as a whole. Even this figure, it turned out, was based on outdated information about minority representation in the borough and more accurate data from the Labour Force Survey and from the Commission for Racial Equality's statistical information suggested that some 48 per cent of the borough's population were from ethnic minorities, including Irish and Orthodox Jewish members. In consequence, a new employment target of 48 per cent was set in October 1986 to be met by December 1990 (London Borough of B 1987a: 4).

These targets, it will be noted, are crude. They are based on overall minority representation in the population of the borough and take no account of availability as measured by age structure, location, qualifications or differential career or job choices. Nor do they disaggregate the minority populations into their component groups, which raises the question of how sensitive equal opportunities policies (and affirmative action practices) should be to the representation in a workforce of each (and every) minority group in the relevant population. Certainly, current monitoring of the workforce in B disaggregates the data into separate groups (of which there is a relatively large number in the borough) but there is little evidence that even current policy and practice is sufficiently discriminating to target different groups separately for equal opportunity purposes.

Equal employment opportunity policy in B

The equal employment opportunity policy of B as it now stands was drawn up in 1986 and remains unchanged despite reorganisation of the managerial structure designed to transform it. The policy statement itself is unexceptional: the council is committed 'to actively opposing racism' (sic); it will combat all direct and indirect discrimination in its employment policies and in the provision of services; it will consider job applicants solely on merit; it will ensure that all sections of the population have equal access to services; implementing equal opportunities will be the responsibility of all council employees and they will receive training to enable them to do this (London Borough of B 1987a: 2, 1987b, 1987c).

There are four sub-components of the policy so far as council employment is concerned. These are monitoring, setting equality targets, providing training, and race-'proofing' all recruitment and selection procedures. Monitoring was first introduced in 1980 and underwent a major revision in 1986 following agreement with the Staffing and Equal Opportunities Committee (SEOC), after which date all non-manual council employees had their racial or ethnic category recorded on the payroll computer, thus providing the means (if desirable) of monitoring ethnic composition at every grade. The successive revisions in employment equality targets have already been referred to but it is worth noting again that, despite the asserted rationale behind such targets that: 'over a reasonable period of time . . . the workforce will begin to reflect the racial . . . composition of the labour market of the relevant catchment area' (London Borough of B 1987a: 5), the baseline figures quoted for comparative purposes remain the crude aggregated proportion of the total population.

The training component of equal opportunities was to take two forms: the provision of a variety of race awareness courses for council staff, and training for members of ethnic minority groups better to enable them to compete in the job market.

Finally, all the council's recruitment, selection and promotion procedures were to be thoroughly reviewed to eliminate any racial bias and this review resulted in the implementation of a number of new procedures and affirmative action practices.

Affirmative action in the London Borough of B

A summary list of affirmative action practices used in B would consist of the following:

- race-'neutralising' all recruitment, selection and promotion procedures;
- monitoring the council workforce;
- setting targets and timetables for the representation of all minority groups combined in the council's employ;
- abolition of internal-only advertising of vacancies (all advertising to be simultaneously internal and external);
- abolition of all word-of-mouth recruiting;
- advertising vacancies in the ethnic minority press. (This practice has been subject to a number of reviews not least because of its apparent ineffectiveness. Advertisements are now placed in the *Caribbean Times, Irish Post, New Life* and *The Voice*);
- race-proofing job application forms – including requesting only information from applicants that is strictly job-related;
- production of job descriptions and personnel specifications with no requirements that are extraneous to the needs of the post;
- obligatory equal opportunities training for all council staff involved in recruitment and selection. (Since January 1982 only officers who have been on this five-day, in-house course may participate in recruitment and selection);
- the right of the Race Relations Unit staff (as well as of the other specialist units) to sit on all interview panels (which, if implemented to the letter, would tie up most such staff most of the time);

- management development courses for minority staff;
- race awareness courses;
- personal development courses for minority staff;
- training programmes under s. 38 of the Race Relations Act 1976.

It will be noted that, to the extent that some of the courses mentioned above are for minority staff (and presumably *only* minority staff), they are pressing at the boundary of 'preferential treatment' unless provided under the rubric of 'special needs'.

Ethnic minority representation in B

Monitoring data allow us to compare the aggregated ethnic minority representation at different levels in B's council over the period 1984–89, but information disaggregated by different ethnic groups is only available for the latter date. Again, organisational change within the borough as well as changes in the way data are presented prevent comparison over time of minority representation in each directorate.

Table 4.2 Ethnic minority representation in B's workforce, 1984 and 1989

Grade/grouping	%/No. workforce ethnic minority (all minorities combined)					% change 1984–89
	1984			*1989*		
	No.	*%*		*No.*	*%*	
Scale 6 and below	630	24.1		1255	49.2	99.2
SO1 and above	103	10.2		468	29.8	354.4
Total officers (i)	733	20.3		1723	41.8	135.1
Total operatives (ii)	840	22.1		1398	32.5	66.4
Total workforce (i) + (ii)	1573	21.2		3121	37.1	98.4

Sources: London Borough of B (1986, 1989)

Table 4.2 shows that there were large numerical and proportional increases in ethnic minority representation in the borough council between 1984 and 1989. Representation in the total workforce increased from 21.2 per cent to 37.1 per cent between these dates, with a percentage increase of 98.4 per cent (from 1573 to 3121). The greatest percentage increase (of 354.4, though from a low numerical base in 1984) occurred in grades SO1 and above. The proportion of the borough's total population that was made up by ethnic minorities in 1985 was 48 per cent. However, this, as we have already noted, is an inadequate basis for comparison, but in the absence of more refined data (including travel-to-work zone information) these figures have to suffice for comparative purposes.

The scale of the increases over this five-year period strongly suggest that the implementation of an aggressive equal opportunities policy by means of a fairly wide range of affirmative action practice has paid dividends, particularly in the borough's ability to extend minority representation into the higher grades. It was certainly the view of the local authority that the increases were attributable to aggressive affirmative action practices. And whilst some of the posts filled by ethnic minority members were section 11 posts and are therefore strictly additional to the council's workforce, their exclusion from the figures would alter the overall picture only very marginally.

C County Council

C County Council has an ethnic minority population that makes up approximately 4 per cent of the whole (C County Council 1989a), and hence lower than the average for the country as a whole. It does not therefore, unlike the London Borough of B, face strong community and political pressures to implement aggressive equal opportunities policy and neither does it have within its boundaries articulate and vociferous interests groups to satisfy. Nonetheless, it has had an equal opportunities policy since 1982, but although this is referred to as an 'active' policy (C County Council 1989a) it could not realistically be called such when compared with the programmes we have already described. Indeed, a report to the Resources Committee as late as 1989 noted that: 'no clear goals have been established which would allow an objective assessment of the success or otherwise of this Authority's achievement of equality of opportunity for women and ethnic minorities' (C County Council 1989a: 1). Only doubtfully can an equal opportunities policy without clear goals or any means of evaluating progress be called 'active'.

Although a headcount survey of the ethnic minority composition of the workforce was carried out in 1984, the first substantive indication of the under-representation of ethnic minorities was revealed by the headcount carried out in 1987 which showed that only 1.9 per cent of the authority's workforce were of ethnic minority origin (compared with 4 per cent of the population of the county; no travel-to-work area data were available). It was also noted that if section 11 posts were excluded from the count, ethnic minority representation fell to 1.6 per cent. Steps were taken in 1989 to give more substance (and more goal-direction) to the policy with a recommendation to committees that 'numerical equality objectives' be introduced and that the progress of the authority's policy be monitored in respect both of employees in post and of 'potential' employees – by which was meant applicants for jobs in the authority. These 'numerical equality objectives' were not called targets (though that is in effect what they were) and the then Acting

County Personnel Officer was of the view that many people in the authority, though aware of the existence of an equal opportunity policy, would be ignorant of the fact that the authority operated targets for minorities and women.

Equal employment opportunity policy in C County Council

In 1988 the County Council accepted the principles of the recommendations of a report by Fullemploy that it should set a target of 'the equalisation of levels of employment between the minority and majority ethnic communities by the year 2000' (C County Council 1989a: 2) and in the following year a recommendation was put to the Resources Committee that the County's equal opportunity policy ought to be more rigorously pursued by means of an Equality Objectives Programme. Equality objectives (targets) were to be set for each department and pursued by means of affirmative action and other practices.

The first task to be undertaken, however, was the production of a personnel database because, although recruitment and selection monitoring had begun in 1988, there were as yet no reliable data on the ethnic (or gender) composition of the workforce as a whole. This was put in hand by means of headcounts and self-classification returns in 1989. The system that was then put in place consisted of the monitoring of the workforce as a whole and of applications, shortlistings, interviews and appointments to identify disparities or areas of under-representation of minorities. It was this process then that provided the necessary information to identify where affirmative action practices might most usefully be applied. Equality objectives are now set for each department (in consultation with the County Personnel Officer) and for 'specific sections, occupational groups, levels, etc. (as appropriate)'. All such targets are set at a level that is deemed to be achievable within an agreed time period, which, whilst having the benefit of being realistic, may induce a tendency to err on the side of caution. Much will depend on how a realistic level of achievement is assessed. In this respect, C's guidelines are more pragmatic than most, reflecting in some measure the availability factors taken into account in US affirmative action programmes. Thus, the following factors are noted as necessary constituents in any attempt to assess what it is 'reasonably practicable' to achieve over a given time span:

- departmental workforce and labour turnover patterns,
- recruitment catchment areas for different posts,
  the ethnic composition of relevant professional and craft bodies (where available, and as a measure of the potential pool of minority ethnic applicants),
- existing levels of minority representation in each department at different grades and in different occupations,

- the level of seniority to which targets are to apply,
- any mitigating constraints such as the need to minimise unit costs particularly in the context of competitive tendering (an unusually candid recognition that there may be a limit to the price to be paid for equality of opportunity).

The targets (or 'equality objectives' as they have been consistently referred to) will therefore vary with circumstance and with each department and section but the potential at least for periodic review of their 'reasonableness' exists in the requirement for annual departmental progress reports to the Resources Committee, the Joint Equal Opportunities Sub-Committee and the relevant Consultative Group. In addition, detailed reviews are undertaken every two years to amend targets if necessary and the affirmative action measures required to achieve them. It is intended that this review process be repeated until 'adequate representation' of ethnic minorities is reached (C County Council 1990: App. H).

Affirmative action in C County Council

The types of positive action used in C follow closely those recommended by the CRE and as defined under sections 37 and 38 of the Race Relations Act 1976, and in consequence carry a heavy emphasis on training. All, or most, of the following are used to varying degrees:

- pre-entry training courses specifically for ethnic minorities (and/or women),
- secondment of ethnic minorities to professional courses of study,
- secondment to other departmental areas of work [presumably to broaden experience],
- post-entry training courses,
- equal opportunities training for all staff,
- targeted recruitment drives,
- race-'proofing' of job specifications and advertisements,
- recruitment of staff with responsibility for ethnic minorities (under section 5(2)(d) of the Race Relations Act),
- promoting the authority in equal opportunities matters (a marginal form of affirmative action).

The annual budget for affirmative action practice, to cover all affected groups and not just ethnic minorities, was £100,000, the bulk of which was to cover the costs of the various courses.

Ethnic minority representation in C

The first headcount of minority employees, as we have noted, was carried out in 1984. The next count was in 1988, six years after the equal opportunities policy had been adopted but *before* the introduction of equality objectives and the more aggressive use of positive action to achieve them in 1989–90. The magnitude of the increase in minority employees both in absolute and relative terms (the latter being demonstrated in Table 4.3) is therefore surprising. Certainly, the increases were from a very low base and even in 1988 minority representation in the total workforce was (as previously noted) 'only' 1.9 per cent as against 4.0 per cent in the population as a whole (and even assuming that labour force representation was less than 4.0 per cent – as is certainly the case, a figure of 1.9 per cent would still denote under-representation). Nonetheless, a total workforce increase between 1984 and 1988 of 4.9 per cent included an increase in the numbers of minority employees of 51.9 per cent (from 499 to 758). Furthermore, five departments in 1988 had an ethnic minority representation that was in all likelihood above that for the labour force as a whole (even though one of these – the County Offices – had seen a reduction in its minority representation). Of the total of minority employees in 1988, 70.2 per cent were in non-manual job categories and 29.8 per cent in manual. The largest single percentage of minority employees (16.1 per cent) were youth workers, followed by teachers (15.2 per cent) and professional/technical/administrative staff (11.9 per cent). Conversely, only 0.3 per cent of minority workers were caretakers and 0.4 per cent firefighters (all figures taken from C County Council 1988).

Table 4.3 Ethnic minority representation in C's workforce by department, 1984 and 1988

Department	% workforce ethnic minority (all groups)		% change minorities in workforce
	1984	*1988*	*1984–88*
Education	0.8	1.1	40.3
Planning and Transportation	0.6	1.1	87.5*
County Treasury	0.5	2.2	300.0*
Leisure Services	5.8	6.4	27.2
Trading Standards	3.5	4.5	33.3*
Fire Service	0.2	0.2	50.0*
Clerk of the Council	5.0	5.2	10.0
County Offices	7.1	5.3	−15.4
County Architect	2.1	1.3	−42.9*
Social Services	2.0	3.8	100.7
Total workforce	1.3	1.9	51.9

Source: C County Council (1988)
Notes: *exaggerated differences due to small numbers
Increase in total workforce 1984–88: 4.9%
Increase in minority members of workforce 1984–88: 51.9%
(Data are also given for different minority ethnic groups but figures are too small to enable inferences to be drawn.)

Table 4.4 Ethnic minority representation in C among applications, shortlistings and appointments, Nov. 1988–Nov. 1989

Ethnic minority group	% applics.	% shortlists	% appts.	% workforce 1987 headcount
Afro-Carribean	4.7	5.3	5.9	1.2
Indian	1.4	1.8	1.5	0.4
Pakistani & other Asian	1.3	1.6	1.6	0.3
Other	0.9	0.8	1.1	–
All groups	8.3	9.5	10.1	1.9
All groups Nov. 1988 – June 1989	8.4	8.6	7.3	–

Sources: C County Council (1989b, 1990)

That the conditions necessary for an improvement in minority representation were being established by the end of 1989 is evident from Table 4.4. Over the thirteen-month period November 1988–November 1989, 10.1 per cent of all appointees to jobs in the council were from ethnic minorities (compared with a representation in the workforce in 1987 of only 1.9 per cent). It is worth noting also that minority representation increased from applicants to shortlisted to appointees and that this was particularly the case for Afro-Caribbeans – though it held for each other group as well. Also worth noting in the context of affirmative action outreach is the fact that even before such practices were given added emphasis (after 1989), the proportion of applicants to the council who were from ethnic minorities was at 8.3 per cent, more than double their likely representation in the county's labour force. If the first hurdle to increasing minority representation is to get more minority applicants, and more of them to the interview room, then clearly progress is being made in C and more aggressive outreach could improve on this even more.

D City Council

The ethnic minority population of D grew rapidly and substantially between 1968 and 1972, by which date it had reached 23 per cent. Growth subsequently slowed but by 1991 nearly a third of the population was of minority ethnic origin, with Asians contributing some 29 per cent, Afro-Caribbeans about 2 per cent and Chinese and other groups rather less than 1 per cent. It was in recognition of this early growth, and the manifest under-representation of minorities in the workforce, that the council adopted its first equal opportunities policy in 1976 – in which respect it was something of a pioneer. The policy was at that stage confined to equal opportunities within the council's employ, though it was later to encompass the promotion of good race relations city-wide. Responsibility for the policy – which from the outset was to include regular monitoring of the workforce – was placed with the Director of Personnel and Management Services. A year after the policy was established, the council began to monitor applicants, interviewees and appointees for administrative, professional, technical and clerical posts, as well as the workforce (*Equal Opportunities Review* 1989a: 15–16).

After six years of operation of the policy there was little evidence from the monitoring data that much progress was being made, in consequence of which a major review was undertaken in 1982 preceded by a few months by the formation of a new Race Relations Unit. There were three broad fronts on which reorganisation would proceed (and which, once established, would form the pattern of current policy in D). The first was the development of a programme of positive action by the RRU and a requirement that each department produce an annual Positive Action Programme – to be monitored by the RRU. The second development was thoroughly to overhaul all recruitment and selection procedures not only to ensure 'neutrality' but, again, to introduce more positive action into the process. Third, equality of opportunity was to be injected into service provision instrumentally through departmental positive action programmes and annually monitored for effectiveness. The policy that was to emerge from this period of reassessment was formalised in the authority's *Equal Opportunity in Employment* statement issued in 1986.

Equal opportunities policy in D

The City Council's *Equal Opportunity in Employment* statement dating from 1982 asserts that the council is 'committed to positive action to promote equality of opportunity' and 'regular, comprehensive monitoring of the results of this commitment' (D City Council 1982). It then goes on to state that the policy would infuse all the authority's dealings with employees and with the public. There is nothing remarkable about these sentiments – they reflect closely those given voice in many another equal opportunities statement. There is a rubric attached to the policy statement, however, entitled 'Why Do We Have a Policy?' and it contains an old canard about equality of opportunity which ought to be nailed (or, at least, pinned): 'Since 1976 the Council has been trying to see that *all people seeking jobs have an equal chance of getting them* and that *all employees have an equal chance of promotion*' (D City Council 1982, emphases added).

We know what the intended sentiment is – that, *all other things being equal*, majority and minority ethnic candidates should have the same chance of being hired or promoted. But that does not mean (because all other things are never equal) that *all people* seeking jobs should have an equal chance of getting them. That happy state can only be achieved by distributing jobs by lottery. Indeed, if every applicant were to be given an *equal* chance, there could be no reason for doing it any other way. If, however, we wish to select the 'best person for the job', then it is to be hoped that our procedures will favour that applicant with a *better chance* of getting the job than anyone else. It should therefore be a cause for some concern that elaborate and costly equal opportunity practices and procedures are set in motion (and not only in D of course) without a clear conception of what the concept means and implies. We shall return to this when we consider the theory of equal opportunity.

The main vehicle for putting equality policy into effect is the Positive Action Programme which each department should prepare annually. This should include details of how the department intends to promote equal opportunities through service provision and in respect of internal employment matters. Most important, in relation to the latter, are the 'equality targets' which form an integral part of the programme. Equality targets were first discussed in 1982 but not implemented until 1985. Though set by each department in respect of its own personnel complement, targets are set for each occupational group, not for a department as a whole. This has clear advantages for establishing representation on an hierarchical basis, but being devolved to departments it can, and does, lead to targets being set that involve very small numbers and very large percentage swings being incurred by the loss or gain of a single member of staff. (It was for this reason that six-monthly reviews of targets were extended to twelve-monthly periods.)

Guidance is provided on how targets should be set by the equality targets team in Personnel, but they must be realistic, attainable and acceptable to departmental managers. There have – inevitably – been differing views within D about how targets should be arrived at. Some hold the view that the council workforce should 'reflect' the communities it serves, but this has more rhetorical than practical force – a shortcoming that is particularly telling when targets are disaggregated to occupational levels. The equality targets team, whose job it is to assist departments in setting targets, acknowledges that the question of availability is a complex one and cannot be solved simply by reference to representation in the city's population. The availability pool for minorities will of course differ for different occupational categories and different grades within the authority. The complexity of calculating realistic availability pools has already been illustrated by the eight-factor calculation recommended in the joint OFCCP/EEOC guidelines in the United States. D City Council has not employed this degree of sophistication in setting its equality targets, but it has gone further down that road than many other local authorities.

The recruitment and selection procedures in D follow a familiar pattern in the manner in which they have been adapted to enhance equality of opportunity. Documents and application forms have been 'race-proofed', interviews formalised, job specifications and qualification requirements amended to avoid indirect discrimination and so on. In addition, a pool of black recruiters is being built up with a view eventually of having one black person (and one woman) on every interview panel (D City Council 1989). Finally, following an audit of the council's race policy by the Race Relations Unit in 1985, mandatory training of all staff involved in recruitment was introduced with an emphasis on race awareness in the interviewing and selection process. One further component of the council's equal opportunities policy – in common with most local authorities that take equality of opportunity seriously – is the promotion of training for minority staff under the provision of the 1976 Race Relations Act to facilitate promotion to higher grades.

Affirmative action in D City Council

D's affirmative action procedures consist in the main of the now familiar batch – but with one or two imaginative additions. The following is a more-or-less comprehensive list.

- the setting of Positive Action Programmes and equality targets within them must both be seen as part of the overall positive action process,
- no word-of-mouth recruiting,
- no waiting lists for jobs to be used,
- all applications must be in writing,
- all posts must have job descriptions and person specifications attached,
- all vacancies to be advertised externally as well as internally,
- all APT and C posts to be advertised in the minority ethnic press,
- advertisements must encourage applications from minorities and should, where possible, contain positive images of minorities,
- each interviewing panel should include a minority ethnic member whenever possible,
- outreach to schools, community centres, etc. to encourage applications and to give advice on how to make job applications,
- job advertisements translated into four languages,
- the recruitment process is monitored, including the use of random checks on records, notes, etc. for manual and craft posts,
- contact maintained with professional bodies to 'monitor' their recruitment processes and the minority ethnic composition of their membership,
- obligatory training in race awareness for all those involved in recruitment,

- the encouragement of black support groups in each department,
- 'shadowing' by minority ethnic staff of more senior officers in their work to enhance promotion prospects (what in the US is called 'mentoring'),
- training of minority staff to enhance promotion prospects.

It is an indication that D City Council takes the 'availability' question seriously that some attempt is made to assess the potential pool of minority members that exists in a number of professions by maintaining contact with professional bodies. This must make a very significant contribution to their calculations of what a 'reasonable' representation should be among architects, engineers, accountants and so on.

'Shadowing' was not a practice that was evident in other authorities. It is fairly common practice in the United States but can only ever have a fairly marginal impact given the numbers of staff involved (and average turnover rate).

Ethnic minority representation in D

The overall picture for D shows a marked disparity between APT and C staff on the one hand, and manual staff on the other. The proportion of APT and C staff who were from ethnic minorities rose from 7.6 per cent in 1983 to 11.8 per cent in 1985 and 17.7 per cent in 1988. For manual workers, however, the proportion rose from 10.7 per cent in 1983 to 11.9 per cent in 1985 but then fell to 7.9 per cent in 1987, to rise again to 8.4 per cent in 1988. A significant amount of the fall between 1985 and 1987 shown in Table 4.5 (a 43 per cent drop) can be accounted for by the loss of minority workers with the privatisation of D's public transport, but not all of it. Minority applications for manual posts remain low and, at present levels, insufficient to make good the loss from privatisation.

That D's affirmative action practices are yielding some success is testified to (at least in the estimation of the authority) by the increase from 12.9 to 34.7 per cent of applicants who are from minority ethnic groups between 1977/78 and 1987 (Table 4.6). Whilst it is impossible in the absence of more detailed analysis to attribute these improvements wholly or mainly to affirmative action efforts, the absence of other significant factors makes the authority's claim at least plausible. Furthermore, the attrition rate for minorities from application to appointment remains more steady in the latter year (nearly 30 per cent of all appointments being of minority group members) compared with 1977/78 when 12.9 per cent of applicants fell to 5.8 per cent of appointments. However, whilst the chances of a minority candidate being appointed (as measured by the applicant:appointment ratio) have improved (from 1:27 to 1:23) they still remain worse than those

Table 4.5 Ethnic minority representation in D, September 1985 and September 1987, APT and C, manual and total staff

	Sept 1985 No./% E.M.			Sept. 1987 No./% E.M.			Sept. 1988 % E.M.			No. and % change E.M. 1985–87		
	APT & C	Man.	Tot.	APT & C	Man.	Tot.	APT & C	Man.	Tot.	APT & C	Man.	Tot.
%	11.8	11.9	11.9	16.2	7.9	12.2	17.7	8.4	13.1	+59.2	−43.2	+2.6
No.	238	294	532	379	167	564	–	–	–	+141	−127	+14

Sources: D City Council (1986, 1988)

Notes: (a) Figures show percentage of Administrative, Professional, Technical and Clerical (APT and C), manual and total staff who were minority ethnic and percentage change in ethnic minority representation.

(b) Between September 1985 and September 1987 the *total* workforce of D fell from 4484 to 4464 – a change of 0.5 per cent.

Table 4.6 Ethnic minority representation in D: applicants, interviewees, appointments, 1977–78 and Apr.–Sept. 1987

Date	Applications		Interviewed		Appointed		Ratio applics:appointments	
	Total No.	% E.M.	Total No.	% E.M.	Total No.	% E.M.	White	E.M.
1977–78	1682	12.9	520	10.0	130	5.8	1:12	1:27
1987	6883	34.7	1850	33.5	348	29.6	1:18	1:23

Source: D City Council (1988)

of white candidates at 1:18. It is worth noting in this respect however that, contrary to the sometimes voiced assumption that affirmative action, unlike preferential treatment, is 'costless' for white applicants, the evidence here is that the improved chances of minorities over the decade 1977–87 has been achieved at the cost of worsening chances for whites – from 1:12 in 1977/78 to 1:18 in 1987. But this, of course, simply reflects a statistical inevitability so long as applicants outnumber posts and non-whites are seen (statistically at least) to be in competition with whites for those posts.

Finally, the overall applicant:appointment ratios for whites and ethnic minorities mask considerable variation in ratios between different grades of APT and C posts. Thus, at the extremes (of grade) we find for S1 posts ratios of 1:27 for whites and 1:29 for minority applicants and for PO1 posts and above ratios of 1:13 and 1:16 respectively. The latter ratios are however subject to large swings, being based on small numbers.

E County Council

The ethnic minority population of E county constituted 4.0 per cent of the whole in 1991 but there was a heavy concentration in the county town, nearly 10 per cent of the population of which came from minority ethnic groups. Despite the relatively low proportion of minorities in the county however, the County Council has developed a fairly robust equal opportunities strategy with an organisationally strong position. What marks it out from other authorities with similar policies, however, is the absence of numerical target setting and statistical monitoring. It would seem that this has more to do with the aversion of the County Equal Opportunities and Race Relations (EO and RR) Officer to numerical monitoring than with any decision made by the Policy Committee or its Equal Opportunities and Race Relations Sub-Committee.

The emergence of equal opportunities policy in E can be dated quite precisely to a decision by the Policy Committee in April 1984 to hold a conference on race awareness and equal opportunities in the county.[3] The conference took place in May of that year with the aim of improving general awareness of race questions and their implications for the council. In July 1984, in light of the conference, the Policy Committee resolved in principle to establish an Equal Opportunities Committee, an ethnic minorities consultative conference and a Race Relations Co-ordinating Unit (E County Council 1987).

It was initially proposed that the existing Equal Opportunities Working Party of Members, which had been responsible for drawing up the 1982 policy statement, be extended to include members of all parties and trade union and community representatives and be reconstituted as a committee of the council. Its prime responsibilities would be to make recommendations to the council on equal opportunities policies (for women and the disabled as well as ethnic minorities) in respect of its role as both employer and provider of services; to advise on the statutory duties of the council in matters relating to race etc.; to liaise with minority organisations; and to oversee the work of the new Race Relations Co-ordinating Unit. In the event, however, final agreement to establish the committee had to wait upon the setting up of the new unit in October 1985. Earlier that year a County Race Relations Officer and an assistant officer had been appointed and these, together with one other new post and three transfers, made up the unit. It was recognised from the start that, to be effective, the unit would have to be functionally independent of other departments, but for resource purposes it would be linked to the Clerk's Department. Its functions, briefly stated, were to advise on all aspects of race policy and to promote good relations between the authority and ethnic minority communities (E County Council 1987: 3).

Though receiving general support at the political level, the creation of the unit was met with a mixed (and sometimes hostile) reception by departments of the council, some of which were antipathetic to the idea of a centralised unit and held reservations about how it could operate within the existing departmental structure. (The county of E is by no means unique in this respect; the appropriate organisational positioning of race units presents problems in many authorities and there is no reason to believe that the reservations expressed by departments in E were not entirely reasonable. Nonetheless, the uncertainty and unease that was created then was to be long-lasting and was to have a significant influence on the development of policy in the county.)

Equal opportunities policy in E

Despite the centralised nature of equal opportunities policies and functions in E rather more effort appears to be directed towards promoting equality of opportunity in service provision than in the authority's employ. Certainly, a range of endeavours are exercised in the latter but in the absence – as already noted – of target setting and numerical monitoring they inevitably look weak compared with the efforts of other authorities. Furthermore, the Equal Opportunities Strategy and Action Plans that every department is required to draw up are virtually silent on the matter of employment, being almost entirely concerned with service delivery.

The language within which the race relations policy is couched is not sparing however: '[E] County Council recognises racial prejudice as a dangerous sickness threatening the healthy development of the human race, and racism as an unmitigated evil of society' (E County Council 1988: 4.1). The spirit embodied in this fanfaronade translates, so far as employment with the authority is concerned, into the following articles of practice:

- that no applicant or employee receives less favourable treatment on the grounds of race (etc.),
- that any qualification requirements are essential for the job,
- to provide training in how to implement equal opportunity policy,
- to assess personal capabilities irrespective of race (etc.),
- to remove all qualifications and conditions that might have adverse impact (because of race etc.).

These in turn are implemented by the usual pack of procedures including race awareness training, validation of tests (though this more in theory than in practice according to the EO and RR Officer), targeting of job advertisements and the 'neutralisation' of all selection procedures. Most of this would come under the rubric of good equal opportunities practice (though there are elements of affirmative action involved). Two points are worthy of note however. The first is that posts are advertised in the authority's 'Job Sheet' before they go to public advertisement (unless they can be filled from the 'At Risk' register of people requiring a job move because of illness or other reasons – in which case they are not advertised at all). In other authorities and institutions this would be considered to be contrary to good equal opportunities practice. The second point relates to the use of the interview.

> The interview should be used as a vehicle to promote the equal opportunities policy and to test the candidate's ability to further the objectives of the policy.
> Candidates who do not display attitudes conducive to the policy should not be appointed.
>
> (E County Council 1988: 13.6)

Were this injunction to be carried out faithfully and to the letter, the clear implication would be that having the correct attitudes is an overriding qualification for employment in E, disqualificatory even of an otherwise excellent candidate. And this is not just a matter of not wanting to employ racists (though even that term has been so promiscuously used as to have been deprived of much of its meaning); it is perfectly feasible for a candidate to have 'correct' views on equity and justice but not to be in tune with the particular methods used to promote them. Furthermore, we know only too well (or should do) how shifting are the sands of 'political correctness'. We shall have reason to return to this topic in a subsequent chapter.

Affirmative action in E County Council

The departmental Strategy and Action Plans constitute the most coherent statement of equal opportunities and affirmative action practice but these, as we have noted, are primarily concerned with service provision. Affirmative action practices are nonetheless used in respect of employment in the authority, but the extent, nature and 'aggressiveness' of these vary from one department to another. Among the more commonly used are the following:

- outreach into schools and community centres often by means of the Ethnic Minority Forum – to spread information about jobs and careers in the authority,
- all publicity material and job advertisements must present 'positive images' of ethnic minorities and 'avoid stereotyping',
- publicity and job advertisements translated into minority languages,
- advertising in the ethnic minority press (with special advertisements for the fire service),
- no word-of-mouth recruitment,
- a review of 'internal before external' advertising procedure,
- in education, the establishment of a pool of black teachers, to enhance the chances of minority group members reaching senior positions,
- validation of all tests,
- 'neutralisation' of selection procedures,
- in-service training focused on ethnic minorities, to improve job prospects,
- equal opportunities and race awareness training,
- identifying the special needs of ethnic minority groups and providing compensatory training.

The list is a fairly standard one and all the practices included are ones that are familiar from other authorities. One item is worthy of comment however – the use of the Ethnic Minority Forum as a vehicle for outreach into minority communities. This would seem to provide a potentially productive method of making contact with the minority population and of learning more about their needs and aspirations. Much however would (and will) depend on the composition and representativeness of the Forum. At the time of fieldwork (in 1990) the Equal Opportunities Officer was of the opinion that meetings with the Forum had tended to be one-way affairs with the authority feeding information to the Forum members but getting little back. Furthermore, the free flow of information has been hampered by divisions or disagreements between the different minority groups and communities (Pakistani, Indian, Sikhs, Afro-Caribbean – and within the Afro-Caribbean community). Such conflicts of course raise broader issues about the value of an Ethnic Minority Forum and the assumption upon which it is based, that there is a community of interests among all minority groups. That there is on *some* issues is undeniable; that there is on *all* issues is simply fanciful.

Ethnic minority representation in E

The guide to equal opportunity (E County Council 1987) notes 'if we look at the current E County Council workforce; black people . . . are not substantially represented and tend to be employed mainly in the lower grades' (E County Council 1987: 14). But, since E County Council does *not* 'look', it is in no position to say that there is under-representation. A total absence of minorities from senior positions is a pretty good indication, but without a continuous headcount *and* estimates of availability for all grades and occupations, it just is not possible to judge the state of health of equal opportunities in the authority.

F City Council

The proportion of F's population who came from minority ethnic groups in 1991 was slightly higher than for England and Wales as a whole, at 6.0 per cent. The breakdown for different minority groups was 1.5 per cent black, 3.8 per cent Asian and 0.4 per cent Chinese or Vietnamese. Although there did not appear to have been any wide-spread awareness of, or concern about, under-representation of min-orities in the council (indeed, until quite recently there were no data available by which to make a judgement) there was, in the early 1980s 'a growing desire on the part of the Council to address equality issues in employment and service delivery'. This led in 1983 to the setting up of the Equal Opportunities Unit which was to cover gender and disability as well as race. Because the authority at the time was without a Chief Executive, and the Director of Administration was designated as 'Chief Officer', the new unit was located in the Department of Administration. Its remit appears to have been unstructured and the unit developed its work without a clear sense of direction so that by late 1989 the council was considering proposals for restructuring it. These deliberations led to a report outlining ideas for a newly organised equal opportunities function (F City Council 1990). This in turn led to the establishment of a reorganised Equal Opportunities Unit which was to remain located in the Administration Department. The promotion of equal opportunities in service provision, however, initially at least, was to remain devolved to service departments (F City Council 1989a).

Equal opportunities policy in F

In 1990, however, equal opportunities policies were not as developed either in theory or in practice in F as in the other authorities we have looked at. Reorganisation was in motion and a more systematic approach was being adopted – particularly in relation to monitoring the work-force and taking steps to increase minority ethnic representation. Much of that, however, was for the future: there was plenty to catch up on in the meantime.

A report outlining a new equal opportunities strategy identified the two main objectives of the policy (and of the new Equal Opportunities Unit) as:

1) To ensure that black people, women and people with disabilities are *fairly represented* as employees in departments of the City Council in terms of their numbers and their grades.
2) To ensure that an effective and equal service is provided by all departments of the City Council to black people, women and people with disabilities.

(F City Council 1990: 23, emphasis added)

Perhaps the principal means by which these objectives were to be put into operation was the vehicle of the Equal Opportunities Action Plan that all departments would be required to draw up. Each plan is intended to cover both employment and service delivery matters, and so far as the former is concerned it was assumed, though not (at that time at least) explicitly stated, that monitoring, target setting and proposed affirmative action procedures would be part of the plan.

Money was voted in 1990 to fund the setting up of a database as the first step to establishing a comprehensive monitoring system. This was to be undertaken jointly by the Equal Opportunities Unit and the Personnel Division and was to consist of an ethnic breakdown of personnel by grade and department, data on applications, shortlistings and appointments, and reasons for decisions. It was to be updated every six months. Departmental targets were to be set (with the assistance of the Equal Opportunities Unit) though no indication was given at that stage (other than the 'fair representation' in the first of the equal opportunities aims) about how such targets were to be calculated. And quarterly reports were to be produced on the progress made by each department on monitoring (F City Council 1989b, 1990: 23, information from interviews).

The *Code of Practice in Recruitment and Selection* issued in 1988 (F City Council 1988) contained provisions for ensuring that no indirect discrimination took place in the hiring process. All of these were standard 'good practice' procedures such as the production of job and person specifications, guidance on how to conduct the interviews, the use of neutral tests (though there is no indication that tests were ever validated) and – perhaps the nearest to an affirmative action procedure – the use of the ethnic minority press for job advertisements. The 1990 proposals were to tighten all these procedures by making the Equal Opportunities Unit responsible for regularly monitoring the entire recruitment process to ensure that all the anti-discriminatory procedures were being enforced.

Finally, in the area of training, the post-1990 reorganisation was to take out such training activity as there had been in the old Equal Opportunities Unit and place it along with all other training responsibilities in the Central Training Unit. Prior to that, most training had been a matter for departments in collaboration with the central unit.

Affirmative action in F City Council

At the time of the fieldwork, affirmative action practices were less developed and less extensively used in F than in any of the other authorities included here. What there was may be summarised as follows:

- departmental Equal Opportunities Action Plans (content as yet unspecified),
- the introduction of equality targets based upon:
  — monitoring the ethnic composition of the existing workforce,
  — the introduction of monitoring of the ethnic composition of applicants, shortlistings and appointments,
  — use of the ethnic minority press for job advertisements,
  — 'equality'-proofing of recruitment and selection procedures, including neutral tests,
- affirmative action training including:
  — equal opportunity briefings,
  — training for recruitment and selection,
  — cultural awareness training,
  — anti-racist strategies training,
  — Section 37 training,
  — skills training for minorities.

In 1990 at least, equal employment opportunities policy did not include therefore any outreach practice into schools, community centres, etc. nor any targeted recruitment drives, mentoring programmes or other strategies to promote minority representation that were in use elsewhere.

Ethnic minority representation in F City Council

A report to the Equal Opportunities Sub-Committee for Ethnic Minorities by the Director of Administration in November 1988 provided the first detailed information on ethnic minority representation by department, by grades within departments, and among applicants and appointees for each department. This was at the early stages of the authority's attempts at detailed numerical auditing, however, and the data were of little value because most departmental returns had approximately 70 per cent of the staff uncoded for ethnicity. The vast majority of these would be white ethnics but the level of under-counting of minority ethnics remains an unknown quantity. Table 4.7 below gives the best estimate based on these data of the proportion of each department's staff who were of Afro-Caribbean and of Asian background. In common with other authorities, no estimates of availability of minorities at each grade for each type of job have been produced and the only comparator is the proportion of the population of F who were from ethnic minorities – which at 1991 was 6 per cent. As we have noted before, crude population proportions provide only a very approximate indication of what minority representation should be in the absence of discriminatory barriers to employment in the council.

Table 4.7 Ethnic minority representation in F, by department, 1988

Department	% employees Afro-Carribean	% employees Asian	% employees Afro-Carribean plus Asian	Total employees (No.)
Administration	3.53	2.07	5.55	595
Education	0.29	0.19	0.48	9965
Finance	2.03	2.76	4.75	290
Highways Eng. and Tech.	1.29	2.26	3.58	309
Highways Eng. and Cleansing	0.51	0.29	0.80	1370
H'sing and Env. Health	1.87	1.78	3.64	1126
Industry and Estates	2.86	1.43	4.29	140
Leisure Services	1.47	0.94	2.42	2442
Municipal Services	1.70	0.47	2.17	645
Planning	0.95	0.95	1.90	210
Public Works	1.10	0.34	1.44	1455
Social Services	1.51	0.39	1.90	8236
Total authority	1.05	0.51	1.56	26783

Source: F City Council (1989b)

Within the limitations of these data, therefore, overall representation of ethnic minorities, when compared with the crude benchmark of representation in the total city population as a whole, is low (1.56 per cent compared with 6 per cent). Only the Administration Department approaches the city-wide figure and the lowest levels of minority representation are found in Education (which may have been particularly susceptible to under-counting) and Highways Engineering and in Cleansing.

THE PRIVATE SECTOR

Agreement was reached with four private sector organisations in Great Britain. They included a High Street bank, a large motor corporation, an airline and a retail organisation. Treatment of these is similar in most respects to that of public sector bodies and they have likewise been left anonymous (though once again to anyone familiar with equal opportunities practice their identity will inevitably be transparent).

JX Bank

Moves to introduce equal employment opportunities in JX 'High Street' bank came in the early 1980s and were partly (though by no means wholly) the result of a threat of a formal investigation by the Equal Opportunities Commission. The bank (in common with all others at the time) was vulnerable on the question of whether it provided genuinely equal employment opportunities for both sexes. The bank reached an agreement with the EOC, one consequence of which was the introduction of an equal opportunities policy which, though having its provenance in gender equality, was from the very start to include race and disability.

The bank's equal opportunities policy statement was first issued in 1985 in a handbook for employees. It comes in two parts:

> The Bank is committed to provide equal opportunities in employment. This means that all job applicants and employees shall receive equal treatment regardless of sex, marital status, race, colour, nationality or ethnic or national origins.
>
> The Bank recognises that most people with disabilities have the same skills and abilities as other employees.
>
> It wishes to recruit and provide equal opportunities to disabled persons according to their abilities.
>
> (JX Bank 1989: 3)

Equal opportunities statements are of course unimportant in themselves and their wording usually carries minimal meaning content (being only 'good faith thoughts'). The section on disability in the JX statement, however, is an example of how, without due care, equal opportunities 'talk' can sacrifice meaning to sentiment. We know what they mean, but to say that most people with disabilities have the same abilities as others without disabilities doesn't express it. It expresses a contradiction in terms.

The first steps to implementing the policy included the appointment of an Equal Opportunities Manager, the initiation of training on equal opportunities legislation and the bank's equal opportunities policy, the establishment of monitoring systems (including numerical monitoring for all stages of the recruitment process, and an ethnic audit of the workforce). The workforce audit and the monitoring of applicants, interviewees and appointees began straight away and the first monitoring results were available by early 1986.

Equal opportunities policy in JX Bank

There are five broad strands to the promotion of equal opportunities in the bank. Three – equality-proofing all recruitment and selection procedures, statistical and procedural monitoring and a variety of training packages – are permanent features across the whole organisation and the other two – outreach to schools and colleges and external training links – are more intermittently and more selectively used.

For JX Bank the provision of equal opportunities is largely a matter of process rather than goals. Producing the right 'climate', and ensuring that procedures are appropriate and monitoring these, is essentially what it is about. The first task, therefore (and what is now a continuing process), was to ensure that all recruitment and promotion procedures were devoid of any indirect discrimination. Instructions on how to avoid discrimination were included in the *Guide to Recruitment Practices* which is sent to every recruiting point in the country. Another training document, *Managing People Fairly*, aimed principally at personnel managers to prepare them for training line managers, lays a great deal of emphasis on avoiding stereotypical assumptions in respect of women and minority ethnic people (JX Bank 1990a). The contents of this training manual are intended to reach everyone in the organisation involved in recruitment but are deemed also to be relevant to all staff whether or not they are involved in recruitment. What the document does not detail are other aspects of equal opportunities such as equality-proofing application forms and tests, the composition of interview panels, or how to 'sell' monitoring and audit to the staff. Like many other organisations with equal opportunities policies, JX Bank adopts the same procedural policies in respect of all the affected groups it considers relevant – primarily women, ethnic minorities and the disabled (though, it has to be said, with some minor variations). The overall practical effect of this, however, in JX's training manuals and guides, is a strong emphasis on employment equity for women to the relative (but real) sidelining of race. The same is true of the thrice-yearly briefings produced by the Equal Opportunities Manager. Most are concerned very largely with gender employment equity and contain relatively little about race. Whilst there are sound arguments for a generic approach to equality of opportunity, the danger so far as consumers (in this case line managers) are concerned is that they will take their cue from what they see to be the relative emphasis placed by the central unit.

Monitoring takes two forms: the periodic appraisal of recruitment and promotion procedures, and the statistical audit of the workforce and applications, shortlistings and appointments. We need say no more here about the review of procedure. The audit of the workforce was completed by 1989 so that by that date the entire full-time workforce had been classified by race and gender. That record is continuously updated by the ethnic monitoring of new appointees (and the deletion of leavers), itself a part of the ethnic audit of the selection process. In general terms, it is expected that the ethnic composition of applicants ought to reflect that of the local labour market (except where the relevant draw area is larger) (JX Bank 1989: 12). This does not, however, entail the use of quotas or even of targets. The Equal Opportunities Manager was of the opinion that what was required in JX Bank was a fairly substantial change in attitudes about equality of opportunity and that the use of targets would not assist in this process. A more productive line of approach, she thought, would be to persuade people that the results of equal opportunity procedures would make good business sense (without any implication of there being a statistically 'correct' result). Even so, in order to be able to identify particular regions in which more affirmative action should be used, there had to be some impression of under-representation of ethnic minorities and hence some 'feeling' for what it ought to be. And that is what it was – an educated guess.

Outreach for recruitment purposes largely entails ensuring that schools with high proportions of minority ethnic children are included amongst those visited by representatives of the bank to give talks on careers in banking. There appears to be no particular targeting of such schools to receive more of such visits, or of any minority ethnic orientation to the presentations. Recruitment advertisements, however, are intended to 'encourage applications for employment from suitable candidates of both sexes and all races'. In addition, advertisements for posts in the bank are sometimes placed in the ethnic minority press, though this has not proved to be a very effective way of increasing minority applicants.

Equal opportunities training at JX Bank takes two forms: internal training mainly for personnel practitioners and involvement in outside training schemes to promote the career prospects of minority ethnic (and other) young people. The particular training schemes are listed under the affirmative action procedures used by the bank and listed below.

Affirmative action in JX Bank

We have already noted that the equal opportunities activities of JX Bank place a greater emphasis on employment equity for women than for members of ethnic minority groups (not of course entirely mutually exclusive groups) (JX Bank 1990b). This no doubt stems from the perceived greater vulnerability of the bank to claims of gender discrimination than to those of racial discrimination. It is not surprising, therefore, that the scope and variety of affirmative action procedures in respect of women have been rather more ambitious than those for people from minority ethnic groups. Affirmative action to promote the representation of ethnic minorities has not, in short, been aggressive. But neither has it been negligible, as the following list indicates:

- monitoring of recruitment and selection procedures and tests and the 'neutralisation' of these in respect of race,
- statistical monitoring of applications, shortlistings and appointments,
- statistical ethnic audit of the full-time workforce,
- some outreach work to schools with high proportions of minority ethnic children,
- job advertisements to encourage applications from qualified minority ethnic candidates,
- advertisements in the ethnic minority press in selected regions,
- equal opportunities awareness training for senior executives and all personnel managers,
- all existing personnel practitioners trained in equal opportunities matters,
- equal opportunities training incorporated into the mainstream of personnel training for new practitioners,
- regular one-week recruitment and interviewing skills course incorporating equal opportunity matters,
- local two-day equal opportunities courses,
- half-day seminars for all line managers on their part in implementing equality of opportunity,
- training managers incorporate equal opportunity matters in training sessions,
- production of a video ('Fair's Fair') used at all levels of equal opportunity training,
- involvement in Customised Pre-Recruitment Training (The Industrial Society),
- involvement in COMPACTS,
- involvement in Community Job Link,
- involvement in the Fullemploy Group,
- involvement in PATH and other local schemes,
- involvement in JIG (pre-employment training for underprivileged unemployed of all races).

Ethnic minority representation in JX Bank

The proportion of staff from ethnic minorities varies greatly (as would be expected) by region and even more so by individual branches. There is, however, as we have already noted, no stated baseline figure used to represent even an approximate target either nationally or at regional or branch level (though equal opportunities policy does contain a general rubric that the ethnic make-up of *applicants* should reflect that of the local labour market). Even the latter is a very crude basis, requiring as it does an assumption that the distribution of people who *want* to go into banking is indifferent to ethnic status. Notwithstanding these caveats there is a big difference between ethnic minority representation in the population as a whole (and an even bigger difference for minority representation in the labour force) and representation in the bank nationally, as is shown in Table 4.8. Not surprisingly the discrepancy (if that is what it is other than purely statistical) is greatest for managers, only 0.06 per cent of whom are Afro-Caribbean or African (one woman and five men) and 0.5 per cent Asian. Of all clerical and managerial staff, 1.5 per cent are Afro-Caribbean or African and 3.0 per cent Asian as against a labour force representation for all minorities of some 4.7 per cent.

Table 4.8 Ethnic minority representation in JX Bank, 1990[a]

	Males		Females		Total	
	% Afro-Carib. + African	% Asian + other non-white	% Afro-Carib. + African	% Asian + other non-white	% Afro-Carib. + African	% Asian + other non-white
Managers[b]	0.06	0.5	0.1	0.9	0.06[c]	0.5
Clerical	1.2	3.6	1.8	2.0	1.8	3.5
Total	0.8	2.5	1.9	3.4	1.5	3.0

Source: Calculated from staff audit data JX Bank.
Notes: (a) All bank excluding overseas divisions full-time staff only, all regions GB.
(b) Interpretation: 0.06 per cent of all male managers are Afro-Caribbean or African.
(c) Male managers outnumber female by 10:1 so per cent female managers contributes very little to total.

Table 4.9 Percentage of applicants attending interview and percentage interviewees offered jobs in JX Bank, by ethnic status, 1990[a]

	Males			Females		
	White European[b]	Afro-Caribbean	Asian	White European	Afro-Caribbean	Asian
% applicants attending interview	24.2	16.7	22.8	25.5	23.8	22.4
% interviewees offered jobs	56.4	51.6	50.3	60.1	20.8	46.4

Source: JX Bank applicant data 1990
Notes: (a) All banks, all regions GB, full-time staff only.
(b) Interpretation: 24.2 per cent of white male applicants called for and attended interview; 56.4 per cent of white male interviewees offered jobs.

It seems likely, on the basis of figures in Table 4.9, that the increased representation of ethnic minorities in the bank will be uneven. Afro-Caribbean male applicants (but not female) have a significantly lower chance of being called to interview than either white or Asian applicants, and female Afro-Caribbean interviewees (but not male) have a much lower chance of being offered a job (20.8 per cent compared with 60.1 per cent for white and 46.4 per cent for Asian interviewees).

KX Motor Company Ltd

KX of Britain is part of an international car manufacturing company with headquarters in the US. The British operation currently employs some 46,000 people at sixteen main sites in Great Britain and Northern Ireland and has had a reputation for its concern over race relations and equality of opportunity for more than two decades. Whilst it also actively pursues job equity for women (and the disabled), it has remained most active, unlike JX Bank, in the field of race.

The company first began to monitor the ethnic composition of the hourly paid workers at its main East London site as long ago as 1967 as a result of which it was found that 34.7 per cent of all job applicants and 32.5 per cent of all those hired were from ethnic minorities (no data were available for the ethnic composition of the labour draw area but it seems likely that, at the very least, these figures more than matched minority representation in the labour force). In 1969, monitoring was extended to all plants in Great Britain when it was found that overall minority representation for hourly paid workers was 10 per cent, the highest for any plant being 34.4 per cent[4] and the lowest zero (KX Company 1989, *Equal Opportunities Review* 1989b: 10).

Although country-wide monitoring was in place, the company was without any semblance of an equal opportunity policy until 1970 and even then it came in the form of a race relations policy that turned out to be but the first step towards a policy of job equity. The 1970 Race Relations Policy is an interesting document for the historical perspective it throws on thinking about race relations and the language in which this was couched. There is no mention of 'equality of opportunity' and the emphasis throughout is on non-discrimination and the importance of compliance with the 1968 Race Relations Act. The production of a written policy (non-discrimination had for a long time been unstated company policy) was occasioned by the new Act but also by 'the increased number of coloured and immigrant employees' (KX Company 1970). The principle of non-discrimination, the policy says, will apply to every aspect of the work situation, including recruitment, selection, promotion and so on, but then finds it necessary to mention also use of the washroom, toilet and canteen facilities. No special treatment, however, would be afforded 'coloured and immigrant' employees who, furthermore, 'should not be concentrated in any particular sections or departments' thus facilitating 'satisfactory integration'. There then follows a proviso which today would constitute at least prima-facie indirect discrimination:

> In applying this rule [of non-concentration] . . . care should be taken not to discriminate against any employees of whatever race or national origin who, by virtue of longer service or other valid reason, have prior claims to consideration for placement in more favoured areas.
>
> (KX Company 1970: 1)

It is always salutary to look back to see how ideas of fairness and fair treatment have changed. What today would be branded by some of the more effulgent sections of the race industry as 'racist' could, two decades ago, be the product of a concern for a balance of fairness to all. We shall have reason to return to this question in subsequent chapters.

Equal employment opportunity policy in KX of Britain

Current equal opportunity policy was established by a tripartite statement issued in 1988 and agreed by the management and hourly and staff unions. Its more salient points (in respect of race) include the following:

> The Company and the Trade Unions are committed to the principle of equal opportunity in employment. [They] . . . declare their opposition to any form of less favourable treatment whether through direct or indirect discrimination . . . on the grounds of race, religious beliefs, creed, colour, nationality, ethnic or national origins, marital/parental status or sex [the subsequent paragraph brings in disability and age].
>
> The Company and the Trade Unions . . . agree that it is the duty of all employees to accept their personal responsibility for fostering a fully integrated community at work by adhering to the principles of equal opportunity and maintaining racial harmony.
>
> (KX Company 1988: paras 1.1, 2.1)

There is much more but it is necessarily in the nature of such statements that, when read in bulk, they begin to seem like a mantra. There is nothing else in KX's statement that is not found in many others.

The *substance* of KX's equal opportunity policy does differ (in emphasis at least) from most others we have examined. Nor is it reflected in the 1988 policy statement in which equal opportunities and race awareness training and skills training for minorities are mentioned near the end, at paragraph 5.1. It is these activities, however, which form the bulk of practice of the equal opportunities policy. The removal of discriminatory barriers within the company is in consequence afforded a less significant position than it holds in other companies and in local authorities. There is a simple (and cogent) reason for this. The head of the Equal Opportunities Department takes the view that the main reason for the under-representation of minority group members in managerial, technical and skilled positions is not that KX is failing to attract them as applicants but that many minority applicants are unqualified. Thus, in 1989, 5 per cent of applicants for apprenticeships were from ethnic minorities but only 2 per cent of the entrants to the training school. This discrepancy led to a validation of the neutrality of the entry tests (which were found not to be discriminatory) and the instigation of an outreach programme to schools. This resulted, over a period of two years, in an increase in minority representation among applicants from 5 per cent to 15 per cent but still a third of these were unqualified even to enter training. The message seemed clear and reinforced the view already held, that what was required above (but not to the exclusion of) all else was pre-entry training that could be targeted at minority young people. It is to this end that the company has concentrated many of its equal opportunity efforts primarily in East London, whence most of its potential minority applicants come.

KX monitors ethnic representation in applicants and those hired as well as in the total workforce (from the hourly paid to managers). However, no availability data are used other than at the level of self-evidence and neither are any targets set. Rather, the main concerns of the Equal Opportunities Department at the statistical level seem to be that the overall representation of ethnic minorities in the company (whatever that turns out to be) is reflected at each grade and that, as we have already noted, representation among appointees reflects that among applicants. (One consequence of the absence of targets or goals is that equal opportunity performance is not built into managers' overall performance appraisal, as is the case in many companies in the US (and a few in Britain). However, in the view of the Head of Equal Opportunities, it is unlikely that this would be done even if targets did exist because of the concern that once goals or targets are built into performance appraisal, they too easily become quotas – particularly if linked to performance-related pay.)

Affirmative action in KX of Britain

Affirmative action measures in KX may be summarised thus:

- provision of assistance with pre-work training,
- Bridging Course from school to entry examination for training school,

- Pre-Degree Foundation Course,
- involvement in Newham COMPACT,
- language training for (mainly) hourly paid employees whose first language is not English,
- monitoring all recruitment and selection procedures,
- numerical monitoring of applicants, appointees and existing workforce,
- in-house race relations and equal opportunity course,
- in-house non-discrimination in interviewing course,
- in-house course on improving race relations at work,
- provision of equal opportunities Open Learning Pack for line managers,
- production of external literature (including sales literature) giving positive images of ethnic minorities,
- all recruitment literature to convey positive images of ethnic minorities,
- outreach to schools and colleges to promote an image of equal opportunity employer.

Ethnic minority representation in KX of Britain

We have already noted that minority ethnic representation in KX plants throughout Great Britain varies from zero to 40 per cent (1991), a range that largely reflects the ethnic make up of the various labour catchment areas.

Table 4.10 Ethnic minority representation in KX, salaried, hourly paid, total, 1987–89

	Salaried		Hourly paid		Total workforce	
	No. E.M.	*% E.M.*	*No. E.M.*	*% E.M.*	*No. E.M.*	*% E.M.*
Jan. 1987	181	1.5	5506	16.9	5687	12.7
Jan. 1988	182	1.5	5436	16.9	5618	12.7
Jan. 1989	194	1.7	5765	17.3	5959	13.3

Source: KX Company (1989)

The ethnic minority representation in the total KX of Britain workforce is shown in Table 4.10 along with figures for the salaried and hourly paid workforces (all plants combined). Representation in the total workforce is high (if judged by the proportion of the total labour force that comes from ethnic minorities) and remained fairly static over the three years. Not unexpectedly, however, there was an enormous disparity between salaried and hourly paid staff with 17.3 per cent of the latter being of minority ethnic origin but only 1.7 per cent of the former.

That this disparity remains so large may well be an unintended consequence of KX's equal opportunity policy which has (in practice, if not in theory) laid relatively greater emphasis on increasing minority representation among the hourly paid workers.

LX Airline

LX employs just over 45,000 people across the whole range of its activities, the majority of whom work at or near to either Heathrow or Gatwick airports. Until 1978 its race relations policy was rudimentary and its equal opportunities policy non-existent. Although there was no ethnic (or any other kind of) monitoring, employment records showed that of the 7000 cabin crew only 40 were from ethnic minorities as were less than 5 per cent of all the other 11,000 customer-contact jobs (*Industrial Relations Review and Report* 1979). (The latter figure might be thought to be a reasonable representation if the comparator is the percentage of the labour force but the labour catchment area for Heathrow – but not Gatwick – contains much higher proportions than the 4.7 per cent national figure, taking in, as it does, the London boroughs of Hillingdon, Hounslow, Ealing and Brent.)

The first move towards a substantive policy came in the form of a Group Instruction from the Deputy Chairman and Chief Executive on 27 June 1978. This drew attention to the requirements of the 1976 Race Relations Act but then went on to outline a policy that was more than a defensive reaction to the legislation:

> LX will ensure equal opportunity in employment for all staff regardless of race, colour, nationality, or ethnic or national origins. This will apply to the recruitment, training, pay, conditions of employment, allocation of work and promotion of staff in all parts of the Company, and at all levels.

> (LX Airline 1978)

An annexe to the Instruction then laid out the new policy in greater detail. Apart from the anti-discrimination components, there were four major areas of concern – the introduction of ethnic monitoring; the equality-proofing of all recruitment procedures, including job specifications, the removal of any practices with adverse impact, test neutralisation, vetting of job advertisements and training for all recruiters; race relations and equal opportunities training, cultural adjustment and language training for minority staff; and attention to career development for minority staff with particular attention to possible career barriers and the reasons for the concentration of minorities in particular job categories. This last point was (and remains) a matter of concern. The greatest concentration of minority employees (all Asian) was in the Catering Services Division where they constituted 67 per cent of the workforce. Despite all efforts since 1978 this situation remains largely unchanged. (It must be open to question how much this is an equal *opportunities* matter. The resistance to change in this concentration owes something to the reluctance on the part of many Asian women employees to leave a work environment which, notwithstanding the tedium of the work itself, is a safe and unchallenging one. If a choice is being made here it must undeniably be a constrained one but it does not necessarily follow that were the constraints to be removed (assuming that to be possible) the choices would be different.)

That there was a need for change in both attitudes and personnel practices in LX at the end of the 1970s is evidenced by the company's explanation at that time for the very small numbers of people from ethnic minority groups in customer-contact jobs. As reported in the *Industrial Relations Review and Report*, the reason lay partly in 'traditional management attitudes that customers flying with a British airline would expect to see white staff only in the customer-contact jobs' (*Industrial Relations Review and Report* 1979). If it had been the case that such management attitudes had been translated into hiring and promotion practices then they would clearly have been unlawful (see Race Relations Act 1976).

Having an equal opportunities policy was one thing; galvanising it into effective implementation was another and this did not really occur until after 1983 with the arrival of a new Chief Executive who brought with him an American perspective within which *not* to have an effective equal opportunities policy was to court, at the least, difficulties and, at worst, some very expensive settlements for discrimination. Even then (and not surprisingly – there were many other pressing matters) things did not happen immediately. A new LX Standing Instruction, *Equal Opportunity in Employment*, was issued in June 1984 over the imprimatur of the new Chief Executive (LX Airline 1984a), the impact of which was to announce that the monitoring of the company's equal opportunity policy would require the recording of the ethnic origins of all existing employees and external applicants and to give assurances about maintaining the confidentiality of such information. The following year the Human Resources Department issued a revised version of the original 1978 Group Instruction on the company's policy on racial discrimination (LX Airline 1985). There were no changes of substance and the policy remained, in its written form at least, much as it had been in 1978. Steady but slow progress was made throughout the late 1980s but policy was kicked into a higher gear in 1988 when monitoring data showing a continued under-representation of minority ethnic groups in the workforce were presented to the Human Resources Strategy Board, established in 1984 to take an overview of all human resources matters.

Equal opportunities policy in LX

Equal opportunities policy in LX has been episodic and, no doubt in large measure as a result of the absence of a discrete equal opportunities unit, predominantly reactive to events and in particular to edicts from the Human Resources Strategy Board (LX 1984b).

Standing Instruction No. 7, issued in 1984, first gave notice of the recording of the ethnic status of LX employees 'in support of LX's policy against racial discrimination' (which appeared to be treated synonymously with equality of opportunity). The following year the Directorate of Human Resources issued its memo which again stated the intention to monitor but also informed managers that they should examine all selection criteria and eliminate any that were not directly job-related, but there remained no overall picture of the representation of ethnic minority personnel in the company. Such a picture first emerged in 1988 in a paper presented to the Human Resources Strategy Board and this paper also outlined proposals for improving what the data showed to be a general picture of under-representation of minorities.

Activity during 1988–89 reflected the expectations laid down in the memorandum of 1985. Monitoring the ethnic origin of staff had continued and 90 per cent of contract staff had had their ethnic origin recorded. A target of 5 per cent ethnic minorities had been set for recruitment of cabin crew for the year 1989–90 (i.e. 5 per cent of recruits, not of cabin crew). Reaction to the data showing minority under-representation had been most rapid in respect of cabin crew (in 1988 only 1.96 per cent of air cabin crew had been of ethnic minority origin) and – ironically – given the earlier explanation for under-representation in terms of customer preference, the pressure came from the perceived needs of passengers, the majority of whom were non-white. More black faces were required in the cabin, not fewer. (It must also be said that the move to increase minority staff among all parts of customer-contact personnel was – and remains – an integral part of a more general diversification of staff to reflect the international status of the airline.) Whether it had to do with perceived customer preferences or internationalisation, however, the move to increase minority representation among air cabin crew appears to have more to do with business needs than a direct commitment to equality of opportunity.

Proposals for the year 1989–90, in light of the continuing under-representation of ethnic minorities, included a reaffirmation by LX of its equal opportunity policy and its promulgation throughout the organisation, the establishment of a 'strategic planning group involving key managers . . . as a means of gaining commitment for co-ordinated action . . . on this issue', and the completion of ethnic monitoring of staff. In addition, agreement was to be sought from departments to increase the number of ethnic minority graduates and pilots recruited into LX and the number promoted to supervisory and management positions. Efforts were to be made to increase awareness of the link between equal opportunity matters and the corporate business needs of LX. Monitoring and neutralisation of all selection procedures was to be continued. And, as a means of further emphasising the international nature of LX, encouragement would be given to recruiting ethnic minority staff not just from within the UK but also from abroad. Finally, a further audit of equal opportunity activities would be undertaken after another twelve months. (Details of equal opportunities activities are taken from LX Airline 1989.)

Equal opportunity policy in LX, therefore, is closely tied to corporate business strategy and the effective driving force is corporate business needs.

Affirmative action in LX

In keeping with the nature of equal opportunity policy in LX, the use of affirmative action (never referred to as such) is piecemeal rather than an integral part of a coherent strategy. The following are the main examples used by the company:

- monitoring the ethnic composition of the workforce,
- monitoring the ethnic composition of applicants,
- monitoring and 'neutralising' all recruitment and selection procedures,
- equal opportunity training modules included in recruitment and selection training,
- setting targets (but only for a limited number of job types – most notably for air cabin crew. The choice of this job type had more to do with corporate image than job equity. There was no specification of methods to adopt in pursuit of targets),
- skills training for ethnic minorities,
- career development for ethnic minorities,
- establishing links with local Community Relations Councils and with schools and colleges (but the latter not specifically in relation to ethnic minorities).

Ethnic minority representation in LX

The great majority of LX staff work in or out of Heathrow Airport which has a large number of ethnic minority group members within its labour draw area (a factor that will be relevant for some grades but not for management, pilots or skilled engineers). And as with other companies, irrespective of their location, it is not possible to say what the proportionate representation of minorities 'ought' to be or what level we might expect.

In fact, the variation between job types in the representation of ethnic minorities in LX is probably greater than for any other company with a workforce in the order of 46,000. Table 4.11 shows the ethnic composition of the entire workforce of LX in 1988 and 1989 (no longer-term data are available) and for selected job types and grades. Senior management in LX is almost exclusively white. The proportion of staff from ethnic minorities in job categories such as administration and services increases from the highest to the lowest grade. The largest concentration of minority group members is to be found in the lowest grade in the catering division where collectively they made up 92 per cent of all staff in 1989, an *increase* of 8.6 percentage points over the previous year.

Table 4.11 Ethnic minority representation, selected grades and total workforce at LX, 1988 and 1989

Category	1988				1989			
	Ethnic group				Ethnic group			
	White	Afro-Carib.	Asian	Other	White	Afro-Carib.	Asian	Other
	%	%	%	%	%	%	%	%
Whole workforce	89.6	1.3	8.3	0.8	88.4	1.3	8.6	1.7
Senior manag.	100.0	0	0	0	99.6	0	0.2	0.2
Admin – all	87.2	1.4	9.9	1.4	84.1	1.1	11.1	3.7
Admin – highest grade	97.7	0.3	1.5	0.5	96.8	0.4	2.0	0.9
Admin – lowest grade	54.1	4.9	37.7	3.3	50.0	1.6	39.1	9.4
Technical eng.	97.6	0.3	2.0	0.2	95.2	0.5	2.2	2.2
Services – all	76.1	2.6	20.4	0.9	73.4	2.5	22.2	1.9
Services – highest grade	84.5	1.6	12.6	1.3	84.2	3.1	13.3	0.2
Services – lowest grade	16.6	3.8	77.1	2.6	8.0	4.6	83.2	4.2
Pilots	99.7	0	0.05	0.3	99.2	0.04	0.1	0.6
Air cabin crew	98.0	0.8	0.8	0.4	97.1	1.0	1.0	0.9

Source: LX Department of Human Resources

The MX Organisation

There are a number of component divisions to the MX Organisation. The largest is the Chain Stores Division with 114 outlets in the UK employing 15,000 people. The next largest division is the Mail Order Division with 9500 employees, followed by the Pools Division with some 5000. A number of smaller divisions including Central Services and the more recently created Credit Data Marketing Services combine to give a total workforce for the organisation of some 35,000. Despite diversification, however, MX remains, and remains known as, predominantly a retailing organisation.

Reputationally, MX has for a long time been in the forefront of equal opportunities thinking and practice and not least because its commitment began long before equality of opportunity had impinged on the personnel profession. In 1965, MX received a complaint of discrimination on religious grounds arising from its longstanding policy of 'kinship recruiting' – of employing the daughters of existing employees (85 per cent of the workforce is female). It was in the course of attending to this complaint that the company realised that it was in all likelihood also discriminating racially. The response was a direct if unsophisticated one – an instruction to all store managers to recruit at least 5 per cent of their staff requirements from the 'non-European' population of the area. This was in 1967, one year before the first Race Relations Act was on the statute book. The recording of recruits' ethnic origin also began at this time. It was, of course, an impractical response, taking no account of geographical disparities in ethnic minority representation in the labour force. Adjustments soon had to be made.

With a long-term history of internal-only recruitment, however, it needed more than an edict to alter recruiting patterns, particularly since the unions were opposed to change, and in consequence little change occurred. And this despite the fact that the son of the founder of MX had been educated at Syracuse University in the USA and had returned enthused by American legislation and practice. In later years, however, he was to exert a strong influence on equal opportunity policy in the organisation, such that it came to be closely associated with him personally.

Further developments had to wait until 1978 when a Personnel Working Party recommended that company policy be brought into line with the requirements of the 1976 Race Relations Act. This recommendation became the basis of MX's policy for the future but only after an interval of four years during which the economic fortunes of the organisation declined and all equal opportunity policy was effectively held in abeyance. During these lean years, however, and particularly in 1978 and 1985 when the company was being slimmed down, the unions obtained agreements on internal redeployment and internal advertising only. These remained in place (and a barrier to real equality of opportunity) until 1989.

In 1983 when the health of the company was improving, and as a means of speeding up the equal opportunity process, it began to develop a detailed Code of Practice. This job was completed in 1985 and the Code was launched as a booklet in 1986. Effectively, this was the beginning of current equal opportunity policy and practice in MX (MX Organisation 1989a).

Equal opportunities policy in the MX Organisation

The 1985 *Code of Practice* was issued in booklet form in 1986, and was designed as a number of check-lists of 'do's' and 'don'ts' under a number of headings. In this form it applies to all affected groups and is periodically reviewed. The Appendix to the *Code of Practice* includes the organisation's Equal Opportunities Policy, the key elements of which may be summarised as follows. The main objectives are to ensure that the 'talents and resources of employees are utilised to the full' and that no employee receives less favourable treatment on morally arbitrary grounds. The policy itself entails that MX will fulfil its 'social responsibility' towards its employees and the communities within which it operates; will recognise its legal obligations under the relevant acts; will periodically review its selection criteria, ensure equality of opportunity to progress and provide training to effect this (MX Organisation 1989b).

A large part of MX's equal opportunity policy is subsumed within this *Code of Practice* (brief details of the affirmative action components of which are given below). Outwith the code but allied to it is a five-year action plan (the Group Action Plan) designed to set and achieve equality targets for each office and retailing unit separately over the period 1987 to 1992.

The objectives of the *Code of Practice* are similar to those included in the Equal Opportunities Policy but with two more specific inclusions – that affected groups are not discriminated against when applying for jobs and that '*within five years* these groups are fairly represented at all levels of management within the Company' (MX Organisation 1986: 3, emphasis original). This is perhaps the most explicit (and ambitious) statement of an equal opportunity objective anywhere in the public or private sector in Great Britain, particularly in respect of race. (It was not realistic however and has not been achieved.)

In pursuit of these objectives a 'positive action plan' was instituted (parts of which subsequently became incorporated in the Group Action Plan), the main components of which were the widespread dissemination of the Policy Statement within the company, quarterly ethnic monitoring, reviews of recruitment, training and career development practices, the setting of annual targets, the inclusion of equal opportunity performance in managers' annual appraisal schemes, and the publication of the *Code of Practice*.

There are separate Group Action Plans for ethnic minorities, women and people with disabilities. The plan for racial equality runs from 1987 to 1992. Essentially, it consists of two parts – a series of equality targets setting the number and proportion of ethnic minority staff for each operating unit[5] and a series of measures, collectively called the Action Plan, to be taken in pursuit of the targets. Separate targets are set for 'zoned' and 'graded' personnel – equating to management on the one hand and clerical and shopfloor on the other. Whilst it is acknowledged that the draw area for management posts will be larger than the local travel-to-work area, however, the same baseline – local minority representation – is used for both. Quite apart, therefore, from the caveats we have already entered about using total local population representation as the comparator, it has to be said that the target figures for zoned staff are likely to be fairly arbitrary and representative of nothing very much. There are other problems over representativeness that are peculiar to a large retail organisation. Large proportions of shopfloor staff will be part-time and Saturday-only workers. Neither of these categories is identified separately in the *targets*. Nor do they take account of the sex and age imbalance in the minority population (let alone in the labour force) nor of the demography of a largely retail workforce. It has to be said, therefore, that the targets have more meaning as applied to the distribution of women and ethnic minorities within the organisation rather than gross representation.

In total, separate targets were set for five sites in the Pools Division, nine in the Mail Order Division, the head office for Central Services, and for forty-five retail stores. Progress towards the targets should, it was suggested, be measured by five annual targets in the following manner:

> 1987 (year 1) 10 per cent of target achieved.
> 1988 (year 2) 20 per cent of target achieved.
> 1989 (year 3) 40 per cent of target achieved.
> 1990 (year 4) 70 per cent of target achieved.
> 1991 (year 5) 100 per cent of target achieved.
> (MX Organisation 1987)

The Group Action Plan was to be the strategy by means of which the targets were to be pursued. Since this is in large measure an itemisation of affirmative action measures, we shall carry over our examination of it into the next section.

Affirmative action in the MX Organisation

The affirmative action procedures in MX can be divided very broadly into the following categories:

1 the setting and monitoring of equality targets,
2 those used in pursuit of the equality targets,
3 training in equal opportunities practice,
4 provisions for minority employees,
5 efforts to create a tolerant multi-racial workforce.

There is, of course, a good deal of overlap between these.

1 • the setting of equality targets (as part of an affirmative action programme),
  • quarterly monitoring of progress to targets,
  • recruitment and attrition monitoring,
2 • advertising jobs in a wide range of media including ethnic minority media and sometimes to the exclusion of non-minority media,
  • outreach into ethnic minority communities as piloted in the 'Fair Recruitment' exercise,
  • use of ethnic minority employment agencies,
  • vacancies for senior managerial posts notified to network of minority agencies,
  • weekly vacancies bulletin circulated to ethnic minority groups,
  • continual review of all recruitment and selection procedures to eliminate racial bias,
  • neutralisation of all tests used in selection,
  • a Code of Practice on interviewing and selection (as distinct from the equal opportunities *Code of Practice*),
  • attempts, through negotiations with trade unions, to eliminate internal-only advertising
3 • equal opportunities training for all involved in recruitment and selection,
  • an equal opportunities component to be included in *all* training,
  • course in managing a multi-racial workforce for all managers and supervisors,
4 • language training for career development,
  • other targeted career development training,
  • continued and expanded use of sections 37 and 38 training,
  • monitoring the take-up of training,
  • mentoring programmes (though on a very small scale),
  • creation of black support groups among employees (a practice that has met with little success),
5 • efforts to change attitudes to race at all levels and to create a more tolerant atmosphere in the workplace,
  • the inclusion of equal opportunity efforts in managers' performance appraisals.

Ethnic minority representation in the MX Organisation

In theory, an organisation with a large number of widely spread employing units with a representation in almost all urban areas ought to be in a better position to reflect the ethnic make-up of the population in its workforce ('reflect', not necessarily 'represent'). So it is with MX: 3 per cent of the total staff of MX are from ethnic minorities, as are 4.3 per cent of the total chain store staff, but more than a quarter of staff in six shops are from ethnic minorities (a gross 'over-representation' compared with the proportion of the local population). The highest proportions are found in Hammersmith (41.4 per cent), Hounslow (38.5 per cent) and in the two West End stores (35.6 per cent and 29.3 per cent). These data can, however, be misleading. In some retail outlets, large numbers of ethnic minority employees are young Saturday-only workers and it is a moot point whether they can be said adequately to represent the organisation's workforce. The information in the following tables shows ethnic minority representation in the total MX workforce and in its most 'visible' division.

A smaller proportion of ethnic minorities are in managerial positions than is the case for whites (5.6 per cent as against 12.1 per cent). More than a third of all minority employees (compared with 19 per cent of

Table 4.12 Distribution of total staff by ethnic origin in the MX Organisation, February 1987

	% white	% ethnic minority
Zoned (managerial)	12.1	5.6
Graded (clerical and shopfloor)	85.8	93.7
Supervisory/technical	2.1	0.6
Total	100	100
Full-time	49.6	47.7
Part-time	31.1	15.9
Saturday-only	19.2	36.4
Total	100	100
Pools Division	17.0	4.0
Mail Order Division	30.0	24.0
Chain Stores Division	49.0	70.0
Other	4.0	2.0
Total	100	100

Source: MX Organisation (1987)

Table 4.13 Distribution of staff in the Chain Stores Division, February 1987

	% white	% ethnic minority
Zoned (managerial)	9.3	3.9
Graded (clerical and shopfloor)	90.7	96.1
Total	100	100
Full-time	35.6	31.2
Part-time	33.8	18.9
Saturday-only	30.6	49.9
Total	100	100

Source: MX Organisation (1987)

whites) are Saturday-only workers, and they are much more heavily concentrated in the Chain Stores Division than are white employees.

Some of these differences are thrown into starker relief when we focus on the Chain Stores Division. Within this division a relatively smaller proportion of minorities are to be found in zoned jobs than is the case for the organisation as a whole. More strikingly, however, a half of all ethnic minority employees are Saturday-only workers and when this is taken into account we find that whilst 4.3 per cent of all retail employees are from ethnic minorities, this falls to 3.8 per cent of all full-time, and 2.4 per cent of all part-time workers. The corresponding figure for all Saturday-only workers is 6.8 per cent (figures derived; not shown in Table 4.13).

Despite the high profile that the MX Organisation enjoys as a progressive equal opportunities employer, therefore, ethnic minority representation across the various parts of its workforce does not reflect unqualified success in its endeavours to achieve 'representation'. An important contributory factor in this appears to be the heavy concentration of minorities in 'Saturday-only' jobs – reaching as many as 80 per cent of all minority employees in some stores.

SUMMARY

The material presented in this chapter is, as we noted earlier, illustrative rather than representative of the kinds of organisation selected. Nonetheless, it is reasonable to assume that the components of affirmative action used by these organisations are in most respects similar to those in wider use. There is a good deal of commonality between the lists of affirmative action and, between them, they include much of what counts as affirmative action at the 'softer' end of the continuum.

We shall not attempt to summarise these data here (they will be used in subsequent chapters) but it is worth reiterating that all four of the organisations described here are, by reputation, among the most active in the field of equality of opportunity and affirmative action. Yet the results of their efforts, as can be seen, are mixed. But so also is the quality of the data we need to draw sound conclusions. Even with organisations such as these, it has proved difficult (and in some cases impossible) to find data that will provide a picture of ethnic minority representation in the workforce over a period of (say) ten years. And it is a consequence of the paucity of such data that it is sometimes not possible to measure the output effects of affirmative action programmes.

5 The real thing
The American way with affirmative action

It should come as no surprise that affirmative action in the United States did not spring perfectly formed from any Statute or Presidential Executive Order. True, it made its first appearance in President Kennedy's Executive Order No. 10925, but only as a rhetorical flourish; it meant little more than desisting from discriminatory actions. Only in the subsequent decade did it become formalised into a pattern of particular requirements that meant more than just not discriminating. It would be quite wrong, therefore, to see the first appearance of the term 'affirmative action' in 1961 as some sort of landmark in the history of race-conscious policy in America. Executive Order 10925 was important for a number of reasons, but it was one step in a journey that had effectively begun in 1941 for purposes that had far more to do with the necessities of the war effort than with any concern for racial justice or equity.

In 1941 America was falling behind with wartime production schedules, in large part because of a shortage of workers. Many of the war-related industries were heavily unionised and excluded women and minorities from the workforce; a large pool of labour was therefore being excluded from a labour-hungry war effort. It was in the face of this potentially damaging situation that President Roosevelt issued Executive Order 8802 which stated in part: 'that there shall be no discrimination in the employment of workers in defense industries or government because of race, creed, color or national origin'. It went on to assert that it was the duty of employers and labour organisations 'to provide for the full and equitable participation of all workers in defense industries'. And the rationale for all this was 'the firm belief that the democratic way of life within the Nation can be defended successfully only with the help and support of all groups within its borders' (all quotations from Presidential Executive Order 8802 25 June 1941). It was this Order that inaugurated the idea of contract compliance which has remained in a variety of forms the principal arena for the practice of affirmative action to the present day. It contained two elements. First that all further contracts between government agencies and contractors must include non-discrimination clauses. Second, it established the Committee on Fair Employment Practice in the Office of Production Management. This committee was partly advisory (to the President and government agencies) but could also receive complaints of contract violation. It did not, however, carry any enforcement powers and some contractors, particularly those that were the sole source for some materials, were able to continue discriminatory practices with impunity. Nonetheless, minority and female participation in the labour force (including contractor establishments) increased markedly during the war years, either in part as a result of EO 8802 or simply because of labour market forces. What is significant is that the progress was transitory. Veterans returned at war's end and reclaimed their jobs and minority and female participation rates plummeted. In 1946 the Committee on Fair Employment Practice recorded in its valedictory report that 'wartime gains of Negro, Mexican-American and Jewish workers are being lost through an unchecked revival of discriminatory practices' (Committee on Fair Employment Practice 1947: VIII, as quoted in Office of Federal Contract Compliance Programs 1984). By 1953, the President's Committee on Government Contract Compliance (the successor body to the Committee on Fair Employment Practice) found 'the non-discrimination provision [in Government contracts] almost forgotten, dead and buried'. Non-discrimination had not survived the exigencies of the war effort. Discrimination had once again become normal practice, a way of life in the labour market. And still, of course, a way of life – especially in the south. *Brown v. Topeka Board of Education* and *Little Rock* were shortly to signal the end of formally sanctioned discrimination in education but the civil rights movement and the long journey towards formal racial equality still lay in the future. But it was at the point when the movement was beginning to develop its strategy of non-violent protest in the face of racial hostility and intransigence that President Kennedy, in an attempt to breathe new life into the non-discrimination ordinances and thus force integration – at least among government contractors – issued Executive Order 10925 (on 6 March 1961) (Presidential Executive Order 10925: 1961).

Although most commonly cited as the source of the first reference to affirmative action, EO 10925 was important for other reasons. First, it required the incorporation in all federal contracts (other than construction contracts, which were added later) of an equal employment opportunity clause and, second, it established a mechanism for enforcing the mandated clause. There is little in the Order, on the other hand, to indicate that anything novel or anything significant was being ushered in with the introduction of 'affirmative action'. The reference to it ('the contractor will take affirmative action to ensure that applicants are employed, and that employees are treated, during employment, without regard to their race... etc.') follows a number of similar adjectival references to 'affirmative steps' and 'positive measures'. It probably entered the lexicon of social policy as no more than a flourish of a drafter's pen in Washington.

Probably of most significance in EO 10925 was the setting up of the President's Committee on Equal Employment Opportunity (PCEEO), chaired by the Vice President and with representatives from all the major government contracting agencies. It was this body that was to enforce the compliance requirements of the Order (Potomac Institute 1984: 11), though primary responsibility for ensuring compliance lay with the government agencies themselves. The PCEEO was also given authority to issue rules, regulations and the necessary orders to implement the Executive Order, and these, for the first time, included penalties for non-compliance, including termination of present and exclusion from future contracts. The emphasis nonetheless remained on voluntary action and compliance and the contracting agencies (government departments) were far more concerned with getting voluntary agreements than with imposing penalties. Indeed, termination of contracts and debarral from future contracts have only rarely been used and this remains the case today.

The implementing regulations of the Order (United States Code of Federal Regulations 1989: Title 41 Chapter 60) also, for the first time, required all contractors and their subcontractors to file compliance reports including statistical returns of minority representation, and the manner in which these returns were to be made became the subject of consultation with the contracting community. This was effected through an organisation of big business representatives called Plans for Progress, formed in 1961, which devised a standard reporting form applicable to all government contracting agencies, known as Standard Form 40. Plans for Progress continued in existence as a rather anomalous quasi-public organisation until the late 1960s.

The next, and most important, Presidential Executive Order (in the sense that it is still the operative instrument for contract compliance and affirmative action plans) came in 1965, but the previous year saw the first tangible result of the civil rights movement – the enactment of the Civil Rights Act. President Kennedy, of course, did not live to see it placed on the statute book but history has proved it to be one of his major legacies. We shall consider the relevant parts of the Civil Rights Act 1964 in more detail in the next section along with Executive Order 11246 and its amendments and the Civil Rights Act of 1991. Suffice it to say here that the 1964 Act covered racial discrimination in voting, public accommodations, public education and employment, and that Title VII of the Act, dealing with employment, incorporates the term 'affirmative action' at Section 706(g) thus:

If the court finds that the respondent has intentionally engaged in or is intentionally engaging in an unlawful employment practice charged in the complaint, the court may enjoin the respondent from engaging in such unlawful employment practice and order such affirmative action as may be appropriate, which may include, but is not limited to, reinstatement or hiring of employees, with or without back pay . . . *or any other equitable relief as the court deems appropriate.*

(Civil Rights Act 1964: 42 USC 2000e–5(g), emphasis added)

As we shall subsequently see, the open-ended nature of the last part of this quotation was soon to be used by the courts to impose remedies for discrimination that went far beyond anything that contract compliance had yet required. Indeed, of the two principal ways in which affirmative action may be required of employers in the United States – that is, by means of contract compliance through EO 11246, and by court imposition to remedy past and present discrimination under Title VII – it was the latter that soon required the most radical action, including the imposition of quotas, which are explicitly discouraged under the Executive Order (though latterly, they have become *de facto* components of many affirmative action programmes).

There was another historic component of the Civil Rights Act that we should record here. The Act also created a new body – the Equal Employment Opportunity Commission (EEOC) – charged with overseeing the implementation of Title VII. Its early years were uneasy ones and it took some time to get bedded in. In the first five years of its existence it went through four chairmen, six executive directors, seven directors of the Office of Compliance and six general counsels (Thomas 1982: 4). Until 1972, when amendments were made to Title VII, it could not itself file suit in court but only conciliate and file *amicus curiae* briefs. Nonetheless, these briefs were influential, as we have noted, in establishing the role of the courts in the imposition of remedies for discrimination.

President Johnson signed Executive Order 11246 on 24 September 1965 (Presidential Executive Order 11246, 1965). Much of its language was similar to EO 10925 (and to parts of Title VII) but its 'bite' was to come later in 1968 with the publication of detailed regulations subsequently amended and re-issued as Order No. 4 and then further amended in 1970 and again in 1971 to become Revised Order No. 4. These regulations spell out in detail what had previously remained a generality about the requirements of an affirmative action plan. The 1970 version of Order No. 4 (otherwise known as Part 60–2 of Chapter 60 of the Code of Federal Regulations), for example, introduced the concepts of under-utilisation, availability, good faith efforts, and goals and timetables, and Revised Order No. 4, which contains an amendment to include women, remains in effect a manual of affirmative action practice detailing what contractors and subcontractors must do step-by-step. We shall look at these in more detail in the next section.

The main purpose of EO 11246 (apart from the subsequent detailed regulations) was to regularise the position of compliance programmes by bringing them formally within government. Thus, the President's Committee on Equal Employment Opportunity was replaced by the Office of Federal Contract Compliance located within the Department of Labor. The OFCC was to have overall responsibility for administering contract compliance and the relevant rules and regulations, but enforcement remained with the individual contracting agencies (Office of Federal Contract Compliance Programs 1984: 12). However, the Order also allowed the OFCC to recommend enforcement action to the EEOC or the Justice Department under Title VII, thus forging the first links between the two arms of affirmative action practice.

Further links were soon established when the EEOC came together with the OFCC and Plans for Progress to form the Joint Reporting Committee whose task it was to design a new standard reporting form which would satisfy the needs of both the OFCC and the EEOC. The new form was first used in 1966 and was known as Standard Form 100 or Employer Information Report EEO-1, which is still (in a modified version) in use today. All employers (and not just contractors) with more than 100 employees, and all contractors with more than 50 employees, were required to report annually on this form the numbers of employees in each of four minority groups and the white majority by sex and by nine occupational categories. The four minority groups were Negro; American Indian (including Eskimos and Aleuts); Oriental (covering broadly Asian and Chinese); and Spanish-surnamed (including people of Mexican-American, Puerto Rican, and Cuban or Spanish origin). (The present groupings are similar but have been renamed as Black, Hispanic, Asian or Pacific Islander, and American Indian, or Alaskan Native (Equal Employment Opportunity Commission 1989a: 5).) Despite the recording of separate minority groups, however, it has never been a requirement of affirmative action programmes, nor of court-ordered remedies, that goals be set for particular groups. Required goals have almost always been for 'minorities'. This is a matter of considerable moment, particularly as in recent years different minority groups have diverged very considerably in their representation in the labour market – and particularly in higher education. It is all the more surprising, then, that the use of aggregate groups for affirmative action purposes has occasioned very little comment or discussion in the United States. This is a topic to which we must return later in this and in subsequent chapters.

The year after these standard reporting procedures came into use and in the same year that Executive Order 11375 (Presidential Executive Order 11375, 1967) amended EO 11246 by extending its protection to cover women as well as minorities, the concept of an affirmative action programme was formally written into the compliance requirements of federal contractors. No longer was it a matter of recording minority (and sex) representation and then, in the event of under-representation, taking some voluntary steps to improve matters. From 28 May 1967, all contractors with fifty or more (sic) employees and having a contract of $50,000 or more were required to maintain and annually review a written affirmative action programme.[1] So were put in place the affirmative action procedures and apparatus that, with some amendments, are still in operation today.

The scope of equal employment legislation and regulations was further extended in 1973 by the inclusion in the Code of Federal Regulations of guidelines for contractors on discrimination on grounds of national origin and religion (including Jews, Italians, Greeks and Slavic groups) and by new legislation requiring of contractors affirmative action in respect of handicapped people. The following year saw similar legislation enacted in respect of veterans. Then, in 1975, the Office of Federal Contract Compliance was redesignated as the Office of Federal Contract Compliance Programs (OFCCP) and was given responsibility for enforcing compliance under both the new statutes as well as for EO 11246. The office has retained that title to the present day.

Not only was the range of affected groups expanding (by the mid-1970s it included race, colour, religion, sex, national origin, age, veteran status and handicap) but also the numbers of government agencies involved and the range of establishments subject to equal opportunity regulations. Apart from government contractors, others subject to the regulations included recipients of government financial assistance in the form of loans, grants or guarantees, state and local government recipients of revenue sharing and other federally regulated employers. This represented a very substantial expansion in equal employment opportunity regulation and involved duplication of effort and a bewildering array of regulations and federal agencies. There was a reaction. Those subject to the regulations expressed, in increasing measure, concern at the plethora of demands made of them and demanded simplification and centralisation of government functions. The Carter administration reacted in 1978 by producing Reorganisation Plan No. 1, which in effect expanded the functions and responsibilities of the EEOC (itself reorganised the previous year) by transferring to it a number of equal employment functions from the Department of Labor and the Civil Service Commission (subsequently the Office of Personnel Management), thus concentrating responsibilities in one body. These new co-ordination functions were detailed in Executive Order No. 12067 of 30 June 1978 (Presidential Executive Order 12067, 1978).

A second important change introduced by the Reorganisation Plan was the consolidation of all federal contract compliance functions in the OFCCP from the original eleven separate federal agencies. This change was effected by Executive Order No. 12086 of 5 October 1978 (Presidential Executive Order 12086, 1978).

One further piece of 'tidying up' – though it was rather more than that – was the production of the 'Uniform Guidelines for Employee Selection Procedures' which now form Part 60–3 of Chapter 60 of the Code of Federal Regulations. These consolidate a number of different (and sometimes contradicting) guidelines issued by different agencies – and in particular the EEOC and OFCCP – and are now used by all federal agencies.

LEGAL AND REGULATORY INSTRUMENTS

Equality of opportunity in employment is determined, enforced and regulated under a large number of federal, state and local statutes and by Executive Orders and federal regulations. Equal opportunity law differs from one state to another. Our concern, however, is with affirmative action and employment equity and this narrows down the number of instruments on which we need to focus. We shall also confine our attention to federal instruments since these, by virtue of their national applicability, are the most important. There are, as we have already noted, at the federal level, two principal instruments concerning employment equity and affirmative action. These are Title VII of the Civil Rights Act 1964 and President Johnson's Executive Order 11246 of 1965 as amended by Executive Order 11375. Of rather less central concern for present purposes are Title VI of the Civil Rights Act 1964, concerning recipients of federal grant and subsidy, and section 1981 of Title 42 of the US Code of 1866, concerning discrimination in the making of contracts. And finally, we shall need to consider the amendments made to the 1964 Civil Rights Act by the Civil Rights Act of 1991.

Title VII

The purpose of Title VII of the Civil Rights Act 1964, as amended, was 'to improve the economic and social conditions of minorities and women by providing equality of opportunity in the workplace' (United States Code of Federal Regulations 1985: Chapter XIV 1608.1). There is nothing in this that (at least by today's standards) is exceptional and it might pass as just another equal opportunities platitude. However, subsequent debate, particularly about allegations of reverse discrimination occasioned by action under Title VII, has necessitated the intermittent reassertion of this principal aim. This has forced the debate in the direction of what may legitimately (and legally) be done to prosecute this Congressional intention.

Title VII prohibits discrimination by employers with fifteen or more employees, by employment agencies and by unions engaged in 'industry affecting commerce' on the grounds of race, colour, religion, sex or national origin. Technically, the power of Congress to reach into industry and commerce across all states stems from its power to regulate interstate commerce. Both 'commerce' and 'affecting commerce' are defined in very broad terms so that, in effect, there are very few types of employers who are beyond the reach of Title VII. Foreign-owned subsidiaries operating in the United States are also subject. The Act was amended by the Equal Employment Opportunity Act of 1972 to extend coverage to federal, state and local public employers and educational institutions and, by the Pregnancy Discrimination Act of 1978, to require employers to treat pregnancy in the same manner 'as any other medical disability' (Equal Employment Opportunity Commission 1986).

The explicit ban on discrimination in the Civil Rights Act appears at Title VII Section 703(a) (as amended) which reads in part:

> It shall be an unlawful practice for an employer 1) to fail or refuse to hire or to discharge any individual or otherwise to discriminate against any individual with respect to his compensation, terms, conditions, or privileges or employment, because of such individual's race, color, sex, or national origin; or 2) to limit, segregate, or classify his employees or applicants for employment in any way which would deprive or tend to deprive any individual of employment opportunities or otherwise adversely affect his status as an employee because of such individual's race, color, religion, sex, or national origin.
>
> (Civil Rights Act 1964: 42 USC 2000e–2(a))

This wording is vague on a number of points and it has been the enforcement agency and the Supreme Court which have, over the years, put flesh on the bones of Congressional intent. Thus, for example, the EEOC has detailed the particular employment activities which are covered by Title VII as follows:

> job advertisements; recruitment; testing; hiring and firing; compensation, assignment or classification of employees; transfer, promotion, layoff or recall; use of company facilities; training and apprenticeship programs; fringe benefits such as life and health insurance; pay, retirement plans and disability leave; causing or attempting to cause a union to discriminate; other terms and conditions of employment.
>
> (EEOC 1986)

Employers subject to Title VII are left in little doubt that its sphere of influence encompasses just about every employment practice they are ever likely to engage in. If the specification of coverage leaves little to the imagination, however, this is not true of a number of other aspects of Title VII and in particular what is meant by 'discrimination' and what may permissibly be done to remedy it both in general terms and in respect of particular findings of discriminatory procedures or acts. As we shall see, the latter has occasioned much debate especially where court-ordered remedies have themselves appeared to contravene Title VII.

Affirmative action and Title VII

Title VII mandates affirmative action in two ways – by voluntary action on the part of employers and as part of court-ordered remedies for egregious discrimination. An essential element of Title VII was voluntarism. In the pre-enactment debates, Congress laid great emphasis on and gave much encouragement to employers to engage in voluntary action to eliminate discrimination and further the intent of the Act. And voluntary action to further the intent of Title VII has always been seen to include affirmative action. The Code of Federal Regulations is emphatic on this matter: 'Voluntary affirmative action to improve opportunities for minorities and women must be encouraged and protected in order to carry out the Congressional intent embodied in Title VII' (United States Code of Federal Regulations 1985: 1605.1). It then goes on to specify the three components of which an affirmative action plan must be made up: 'An affirmative action plan or program under this section [1608.4] shall contain three elements: a reasonable self analysis: a reasonable basis for concluding action is appropriate: and reasonable action' (United States Code of Federal Regulations 1985: 1608.4). The prescriptive details of how an affirmative action plan is to be implemented are then provided in the Uniform Guidelines which, as we have noted, apply equally to affirmative action under EO 11246.

Throughout the 1980s and into the 1990s voluntary affirmative action has been increasingly undertaken by companies under Title VII and modelled on the Uniform Guidelines (United States Code of Federal Regulations 1989 60–3.13 and 60–3.17). However, it cannot be said that all, or even much, of this activity has been carried out in pursuit of Congressional intent behind Title VII. It has been, in very large measure, an insurance policy against the day that a company may find itself in court facing a discrimination claim the consequences of which, if found guilty, may well be very costly, particularly in terms of back-pay liabilities (see Bowser 1989). Having a voluntary affirmative action plan in place will not insulate a company from charges of discrimination but it will demonstrate good faith efforts and in all likelihood reduce the damage.

What has proved to be of greater concern, and the cause of much contention, has been the use of affirmative action under Title VII by the courts for the purposes of judicial relief. We shall examine the debate about the protection from reverse discrimination charges of Title VII remedial action in a later chapter (along with a number of other contentious matters raised by the practice of affirmative action), and our purpose here is simply to record the scope that Title VII affords for the imposition of affirmative action for remedial purposes. The relevant part of Title VII, as we have seen, asserts that the court may, in the instance of a finding of unlawful employment practices, 'order such affirmative action as may be appropriate' and that this may include, but need not be limited to, reinstatement, hiring (of an employee unlawfully denied employment), the use of back pay 'or any other equitable relief as the court deems appropriate' (Civil Rights Act 1964: 42 United States Code 2000e–2(j)). The Federal Courts of Appeals were, within seven years, to deem appropriate the remedial use of fixed goals for minorities[2] (which others deemed to be quotas) and though by 1981 nine such cases had been upheld, the question of whether such court-imposed goals/quotas themselves contravened Title VII was one that would eventually force itself on the Supreme Court in *Firefighters Local 1785 v. Stotts* (1984) (467 US 561), of which more anon.

The Griggs Doctrine

Six years after the Civil Rights Act became effective (in 1965), the Supreme Court heard *Griggs v. Duke Power Co.* (1971), which had a greater impact on employment equity practice than any other case to come before the Court. *Griggs* was the first major Title VII case to come before the Court and its recognition of consequence as well as intent as adequate grounds for a finding of unlawful discrimination opened the way to whole-class remedies and thence to affirmative action, first as a remedial practice and then as prophylactic.

Prior to the *Griggs* opinion, handed down by a unanimous Court, a finding of discrimination depended on a showing of intent to discriminate either overtly or covertly. And proving intent is a notoriously difficult thing to do other than in the most blatant cases. It was of the utmost significance, therefore, that the Supreme Court decided that practices which were facially non-discriminatory and pursued without intent to discriminate but which nonetheless had a disproportionate impact on one racial group compared with another were, within the meaning of Title VII, discriminatory.

Duke Power Co. had openly discriminated against blacks prior to the effective date of Title VII by limiting them to the worst manual jobs from which there was no possibility of promotion. When Title VII became effective the explicitly discriminatory practices were replaced by a stipulation that progression out of these jobs required either a high school diploma or a successful score on two ability tests.[3] These requirements were such that the chances of black employees progressing out of the worst jobs were severely curtailed because they were much less likely to have a high school diploma and, as a group, scored less well on the aptitude tests. The effect, therefore, was to perpetuate the pre-Title VII situation. Furthermore, Duke Power had not shown (or attempted to show) that the tests it was using were predictive of better performance on whatever jobs might be progressed to.

What was at issue so far as the Court was concerned was the following:

> whether an employer is prohibited [by Title VII] from requiring a high school education or passing of a standardised general intelligence test as a condition of employment in or transfer to a job when: a) neither standard is shown to be significantly related to successful job performance, b) both requirements operate to disqualify Negroes at a substantially higher rate than white applicants, and c) the jobs in question formerly had been filled only by white employees as part of a long-standing practice of giving preference to whites.
>
> (*Griggs v. Duke Power Co.* 1971 401: US at 425–6)

There are a number of strands to the question and to the way in which the Supreme Court decided it. Indeed, in some respects Chief Justice Burger's opinion (on behalf of all the Court) is both contrary and confusing and *Griggs* is, as Belton has noted, 'perhaps a legal centrepiece of major internal contradictions' (Belton 1981: 542). What is most significant in *Griggs* is the grounds on which the Supreme Court did *not* decide the questions above. First, it must have been open to the Court to decide the case on grounds of intent. Though the tests were facially neutral, the company must have known that they would in effect serve to filter out blacks and indeed they were introduced for this very purpose. In other words, there was in all likelihood an intent to continue past discrimination by means of different practices. The Court did not pursue this line of argument. Second, the Court considered the matter of prior discrimination and whether this might be grounds for a finding:

> Under the [Civil Rights] Act, practices, procedures or tests neutral on their face, and even neutral in terms of intent, cannot be maintained if they operate to 'freeze' the *status quo* of prior discriminatory employment practices.
>
> (*Griggs v. Duke Power* 1971: 401 US at 429–30)

Now, as Belton notes, had the Court relied solely on the issue of facially neutral practices 'freezing' the effects of prior discrimination, then in the absence of any prior discrimination it is quite possible that it would have found the tests valid (there being nothing to 'freeze') and the birth of the idea of indirect discrimination and adverse impact would have had to await another day (see Belton 1981: 543). All the more important, therefore, is the fact that the Court did not rely solely on a finding of prior discrimination and were thus enabled to find that facially neutral tests could be discriminatory in and of themselves.

Nevertheless, it could not have been the intention of the framers of Title VII that all tests which had a disparate impact must be deemed unlawful, because this could well include tests that *were* necessary because diagnostic of job performance. The proviso was, therefore, that non-neutral tests would be unlawful *unless* related to job performance and necessary for the prosecution of business:

> The Act proscribes not only overt discrimination but also practices that are fair in form but discriminatory in operation. The touchstone is business necessity. If an employment practice which operates to exclude Negroes cannot be shown to be related to job performance, the practice is prohibited.
>
> (*Griggs v. Duke Power* 1971: 401 US at 431)

The Supreme Court found that Duke Power had not demonstrated that the tests were predictive of job performance or that they were necessary for the proper conduct of the business. The use of the tests was deemed unlawful and the Supreme Court wrote into the history of employment equity practice the idea of 'disparate impact' as a form of discrimination alongside 'disparate treatment'. This idea of disparate impact without validation of business necessity became known as the Griggs Doctrine and, as we have noted, opened the way for a new range of discrimination charges and for the practice of affirmative action.

It is important to emphasise once again that after *Griggs* the two types of discrimination – disparate treatment and disparate impact – were quite separate entities and that although the Supreme Court did not satisfactorily settle the issue of intent, it is not necessary in a disparate impact case to show intent (see Bowser 1990: 3–7).

It is reasonable to say that the Griggs Doctrine has given rise to a new dimension in employment practice and that much of the affirmative action apparatus now in place for measuring availability and utilisation and the monitoring of goals and timetables, let alone validating tests for business necessity and neutral effect, is entirely dependent on the concept of disparate impact. (It is also worth noting that the *Griggs* decision influenced the drafters of the Race Relations Act 1976 in Great Britain in their formulation of the idea of 'indirect discrimination' (see Pearn 1978: 8).)

Griggs required the development of an entirely new body of case law and as the courts and the EEOC went to work in this uncharted territory, it soon became apparent that disparate impact was going to be charged not only in respect of tests and qualifications, but across a range of other practices too. Levin-Epstein notes the following examples (among others):

- a refusal to hire job applicants because of their arrest record (*Gregory v. Litton Systems Inc.* 1972, *Green v. Missouri Pacific Railroad* 1975),
- word-of-mouth recruiting in predominantly white institutions (*United States v. Georgia Power* 1973),

- refusal to employ applicants because of their poor credit record (EEOC Decision No. 72–0427 1972),
- preferential hiring of relatives in predominantly white establishments (EEOC Decision No. 71–797 1971),
- use of minimum height requirement (*Dothard v. Rawlinson* 1977, *Davis v. County of Los Angeles* 1976).

(see Levin-Epstein 1987: 90–91)

The ban by the New York Transit Authority on the employment of methadone users however was, as we have noted, deemed to fall within the 'business necessity' standard and upheld.

There are two subscripts to *Griggs* that we should note at this stage. The first represents a development of the doctrine, the other, a partial reversal. In 1975 the Supreme Court decided *Albermarle Paper Co. v. Moody* (1975) which established the idea of 'make-whole' relief. This entailed a broad reading of Title VII Section 706(g) ('any other equitable relief as the court deems appropriate') and established the principle that victims of discrimination, whether intentional or un-intentional, should, by way of remedy, be (re)instated to the position they would have held (including back pay, benefits, etc.) had the discrimination not occurred. This, combined with the Griggs Doctrine of adverse impact, established the pattern of remedial action for years to come. Furthermore, a disparate impact finding had the potential to involve a large number of victims and the costs of providing make-whole remedy to all of them could involve a company in very heavy financial costs. Voluntary affirmative action programmes as insurance against such an eventuality began to look all the more attractive.

The year 1989 saw a number of important decisions by the Supreme Court on affirmative action and related matters. All have been inter-preted as inimical to affirmative action (and civil rights) both in letter and in spirit, and it was in an attempt to reinstate what they had apparently struck down that two civil rights bills were submitted to Congress in 1990/91. We shall have more to say about these Supreme Court decisions and the tortuous progress towards the Civil Rights Act 1991 subsequently, but one of the decisions is relevant to the present discussion because it appears to haul in the reins on the Griggs Doctrine, the case involving Ward's Cove Packing Co. canned salmon in Alaska. The bulk of the low-skilled, low-paying jobs in the cannery were held by non-whites, including numbers of Aleut hired on a seasonal basis. The bulk of both skilled and unskilled higher-paying non-cannery jobs were held by whites. In 1972 minority employees filed suit that Ward's Cove's hiring and promotion procedures were dis-criminatory and this was upheld by the Ninth Circuit Court. This and intervening findings were reversed by the Supreme Court in 1989 in a split (5–4) decision entailing what have been seen as three shifts away from the spirit of and acknowledged practice under the Griggs Doctrine. Of greater importance was the Court's dilution of the 'business necessity' test to one of 'substantial service of legitimate employer goals' (*Ward's Cove Packing Co. v. Atonio* 1989). This made it much easier for an employer to 'validate' a discriminatory test (see Murphy 1989). Second, in what some have seen as an assault on the spirit of *Griggs*, the Court shifted the burden of proving disparate impact from the employer to the employee. Furthermore, it was no longer adequate to demonstrate that hiring and promotion practices *in general* had a disparate impact; the employee was faced with the much more difficult task (requiring access to materials held by the employer) of identifying *particular* practices that had this effect (see Murphy 1989, Goldstein 1989, but see also St Antoine 1989, who maintains that the burden of proof has always lain with the plaintiff).

It was as much to reinstate these aspects of the Griggs Doctrine as anything else that the compromise 1991 Civil Rights Act entered the statutes, though, in order to preserve the brittle network of alliances necessary to ensure its passage, the language of the Bill had to remain so vague in parts as still to leave much to the courts to decide. Neither will the Act bring relief to the minority employees of Ward's Cove; Title IV Section 402b of the Act states that nothing in the Act 'shall apply to any disparate impact case for which a complaint was filed before March 1, 1975, and for which an initial decision was rendered after October 30, 1983'. These datelines are carefully set to include only one case – *Ward's Cove*. The patchwork of petty concessions and gains necessary to get the Act through Congress and over another[4] potential Presidential veto are all too clear.

Title VI

Title VI of the Civil Rights Act has similar intent to Title VII but is addressed to institutions and establishments that are in receipt of financial grant or assistance from the federal government rather than to federal contractors. Title VI holds that:

> No person in the United States shall, on the ground of race, color or national origin, be excluded from participation in, be denied of the benefits of, or be subjected to discrimination under any program or activity receiving Federal financial assistance.
>
> (United States Code 1976: 42 USC section 2000d)

Though the vast majority of employment equity and affirmative action cases are brought under Title VII, Title VI brings under the same umbrella institutions that are not strictly federal contractors. Thus, almost all universities will be in receipt of federal assistance of some kind and will in consequence be subject to the same requirements as contractors under Title VII. It is for this reason that the landmark *Bakke* case was decided partly on Title VI grounds (and partly under the Equal Protection Clause of the 14th Amendment) (*Regents of the University of California v. Bakke* 1978).

Executive Order 11246

The purpose of Executive Order 11246 as amended by Executive Order 11325 (hereafter EO 11246) is similar to that of Title VII: 'to improve the economic and social conditions of minorities . . . by providing equality of opportunity in the workplace'. The key difference between the two, however, is that the former is a regulatory programme that does not have the firm statutory basis of Title VII (Organisation Resource Counselors Inc. 1984: 7).

There are three federal agencies involved in monitoring the employment equity and affirmative action efforts of federal contracts – the Office of Federal Contract Compliance Programs, the Equal Employment Opportunities Commission, and the US Department of Justice, but the first of these plays by far the largest part in overseeing the implementation of EO 11246. The Executive Order itself lays down the general principles of non-construction contractors' agreements (EO 11246 Part II B)[5] but the detailed requirements are laid down in the US Code of Federal Regulations (1989: Chapter 60) the purpose of which is to achieve the aims of the relevant parts of the Executive Order. The basic requirements of the Executive Order are first, that federal contractors having contracts or subcontracts with the government in excess of $10,000 must comply with the non-discrimination requirements of the order – that is, to refrain from discriminating against any employee or job applicant on the grounds of race, colour, religion, sex or national origin, and second (and of much greater significance) that contractors or subcontractors with a contract of $50,000 or more *and* having fifty or more employees must, as well as desisting from discrimination, take the following action:

- prepare an annual written affirmative action programme (AAP) to ensure non-discrimination, to monitor the workforce composition, and in the event of the under-utilisation of minorities or women, prepare a plan to correct any imbalance, including the setting of goals and timetables;
- state their equal opportunity commitment in all job advertisements;
- advise all labour unions with which they deal of the commitments under the Order;
- include all the obligations under the Order in any subcontract they enter into;

- allow access to all materials that might be relevant to establishing whether they are complying;
- file regular compliance reports with the OFCCP.

In this section our main concern will be with the nature of affirmative action practices under EO 11246 and with the contents of an affirmative action programme but before that it is necessary to fill in more of the background concerning the role of the OFCCP. This can be done briefly. First, on the magnitude of the enterprise, the OFCCP oversees some 215,000 federal contractors (including construction contractors) and the Executive Order regulations cover more than 30 million workers. The dollar value of contracts covered by EO 11246 regulations in 1987 was in excess of $167 billion (Cooper 1987: VII). The sweep of the Executive Order is clearly very broad and takes in the majority of the 'Fortune 500' companies in the United States. Clearly, it would require massive resources in money and manpower comprehensively to police this size of operation. The OFCCP is abundant in neither. Indeed the number of staff in the Office has fallen from 1500 nationwide in 1978 when contract compliance responsibility was consolidated in it, to 970 in 1990 largely as a result of the deregulatory measures during the Reagan administration. At this level of staffing, it has been said by one of its regional directors to be operating at no more than a minimal level of effectiveness (interview, Regional Director (Philadelphia)).

In the broadest of terms, the role of the OFCCP is to see that the requirements of EO 11246 are being fulfilled by contractors, but it sees its function to include the more positive job of advising, helping and encouraging also. Nonetheless, policing is what must preoccupy the office given the size of the task and the diminutive size of its staff. Policing is conducted primarily by means of compliance reviews and companies may be selected for review as a result of a failure to correct previously identified under-utilisation, a pattern of complaints about discrimination or, more generally, by a process of regular selection based upon comparisons of minority representation in similar types of company in the same labour market area. The base data for these comparisons are derived from the standard reporting form EE0-1. (Before 1983, the selection of companies for review was both haphazard and arbitrary and the present, more systematic comparative exercise was adopted after a company in New Orleans sued the OFCCP for unwarrantedly being subjected to review.) A compliance review involves a detailed and painstaking examination of a company's entire personnel procedures. In addition to these triggers for a compliance review, all contractors and known subcontractors bidding for contracts of $1 million or more are subject to a pre-award review. Finally, by way of its immediate policing function, the OFCCP may receive complaints of discrimination, though complaints under the Executive Order alleging individual discrimination are normally referred to the EEOC, whilst the OFCCP deals with class-wide discrimination complaints.

When a violation of EO 11246 has been identified, or a deficiency in respect of an affirmative action programme come to light, the first response of the OFCCP is to seek a remedy or compliance by negotiation and conciliation. This is always the preferred method rather than immediate recourse to legal remedy. If this fails, sanctions may be imposed in an attempt to persuade a company into compliance. In seeking voluntary remedies, the OFCCP will enter into agreements with the 'offending' company which will provide for remedial action to correct for violations which have come to light as a result of a complaints investigation. Such remedial action might include (where appropriate) the award of back pay and benefits, 'front pay' where a complaint victim cannot immediately be hired, and retroactive seniority. Where deficiencies in an affirmative action programme or its implementation have come to light as the result of a compliance review, the OFCCP will again enter into agreements covering amendments to the programme (such as new goals and timetables) and renewed attempts to show good faith efforts in working towards the goals – which in most cases will require quite specifically laid down courses of action. If, however, in the case of persistent violation or deficiencies, sanctions are applied, this will be effected through the Secretary of Labor of whose department the OFCCP is a part.[6] The Secretary of Labor is authorised in such cases, and where appropriate, to cancel, terminate or suspend a contract or part of a contract, or to render a company ineligible for consideration for future contracts. In practice, however, these sanctions are very rarely used and it remains the policy of OFCCP wherever possible to achieve a remedy by conciliation and agreement. If conciliation and sanctions fail and this is accompanied by egregious discriminatory behaviour, the OFCCP may, as we have already noted, refer a case to the EEOC or the Department of Justice.

Affirmative action and Executive Order 11246

The required components of an affirmative action programme for contractors with fifty employees or more and a federal contract of $50,000 or more are laid down in Chapter 60 of the Code of Federal Regulations, Part 60.2 (otherwise known as Revised Order No. 4). Such contractors are required to develop an affirmative action programme for *each* establishment. Though the company as a whole may therefore have large proportions of affected groups, it may be required to take remedial steps at any and every local plant that is shown to be under-utilising minorities. According to Revised Order No. 4, an affirmative action programme is 'a set of specific and result-oriented procedures to which a contractor commits itself to apply every good faith effort. The objective of these procedures plus such efforts is equal employment opportunity' (United States Code of Federal Regulations 1989: 41 CFR 60–2.10). The regulations also seek to emphasise the mutual reinforcement of procedures and good faith efforts within the programme: 'Procedures without effort to make them work are meaningless; and effort, undirected by specific and meaningful procedures, is inadequate' (United States Code of Federal Regulations 1989: 41 CFR 60–2.10).

The principal components of an affirmative action programme as detailed in Revised Order No. 4 are as follows.[7]

- *Workforce analysis* – an analysis by every job title (or identifiable job type) of the workforce in terms of each affected group, whites and by sex.
- *Availability analysis*[8] – an analysis of the numbers and percentages of each affected group who are 'available' for work in each job title. 'Available' in this context means living within the labour draw area for each job title,[9] being available for work and being qualified or being capable of being trained up to qualification for a job under the relevant job title. The regulations list eight factors that may be taken into account in calculating availability, though a contractor is not required to use all eight. The eight factors differ for minorities and women. The list below is that for minorities:

    the minority population in the labour draw area of a facility,

    the size of the minority unemployment force in the draw area,

    the percentage of the total workforce in the draw area that is minority,

    the availability of minorities having the requisite skills in the draw area,

    the availability of minorities with requisite skills in an area from which the contractor could reasonably recruit (which may be more extensive than the immediate draw area),

    the availability of promotable and transferable minorities within the organisation,

    the existence of training institutions capable of training persons in the requisite skills,

    the amount of training that the contractor can reasonably undertake to make all job types available to minorities.[10]

    (Derived from United States Code of Federal Regulations 1989: 41 CFR 60–2.11(b)(1) (i)–(vii)

The contractor must derive from a combination of all or some of these indicators an assessment of the numbers and percentages of each minority group who might reasonably be expected to be available for work in the facility. This availability figure is then taken to be an approximation of the numbers and percentages of minorities that ought to be found in each job type if minorities are 'fully utilised'.

- *Utilisation analysis* – an estimate of the extent, if any, of the under-'representation' of minorities in any given job category based on a comparison of the workforce analysis and the availability analysis. (These separate steps to the analysis are not identified in Revised Order No. 4; they are specified here for the sake of clarity.) 'Under-utilisation', which in most circumstances will trigger an affirmative action *plan* (active policies to increase minority representation), is defined in the regulations as: 'having fewer minorities or women in a particular job group than would reasonably be expected by their availability' (United States Code of Federal Regulations 1989: 41 CFR 60–2.11(b)).

No particular method of calculating under-utilisation is provided in the regulations and contractors are thus allowed a degree of flexibility in deciding at what point a difference between availability and current representation constitutes under-utilisation. A commonly used measure is the '80 per cent rule'[11] by which a minority is deemed to be under-utilised if its presence in a job category is less than 80 per cent of availability. Alternatively, a contractor may decide that anything less than 100 per cent of availability represents under-utilisation. Whatever the method used, however, it will be subject to scrutiny by the OFCCP (see Cooper 1987: 9.26).

- *Establishment of goals and timetables* – In the event that under-utilisation of minorities is found in any given job category, the contractor is required to take steps to reduce and erase such under-utilisation by a variety of measures. The first step is to set goals for the proportion of each job category that should be held by minority employees. These goals are set annually by the contractor (not by the OFCCP) and will normally be equal to the availability percentage for the given job category. Numerical goals are not required. Though the preceding analyses are broken down by each minority group, the percentage goals, as we have already noted, are set for all minorities combined. Thus, there will not normally be separate goals for blacks, Hispanics, Asian-Americans and so on, even though, as we shall see, inter-minority group differences are assuming an increasing importance not only in respect of affirmative action but also in the context of race policies more generally. The OFCCP may, however, in exceptional circumstances require goals to be set in respect of a particular minority group if it finds that that group is substantially under-utilised in comparison with other groups. (United States Code of Federal Regulations 1989:41 CFR 60–2.12 (1)).

Revised Order No. 4 makes a number of other stipulations about goals and timetables both by way of guidance and warning. They should be realistic in the sense of being 'attainable' in the context of the under-utilisation analysis and by 'putting forth every good faith effort'. The goals should be 'significant, measurable, and attainable' and be 'specific for planned results, with timetables for completion'. They must be designed 'to correct any identifiable deficiencies' and must take account of 'anticipated expansion, contraction and turnover of and in the workforce'. And, of greatest significance, with the benefit of hindsight, the regulations proscribe the idea of using quotas: 'Goals may not be rigid and inflexible quotas which must be met, but must be targets reasonably attainable by means of applying every good faith effort to make all aspects of the entire affirmative action program work' (United States Code of Federal Regulations 1989: 41 CFR 60–2.12(e)). It is a proscription that many would claim has gone unheard and unheeded. Certainly, the question of goals versus quotas, far from subsiding in recent years, has developed into probably *the* main issue in race relations in America. We shall examine this debate in Chapter 8.

The regulations then go on to note a range of other components of an affirmative action programme but the ones we have outlined above constitute by far the main items. The 'additional required ingredients' of a programme (but to which it need not necessarily be limited) consist of the following:

- the development or reaffirmation of an equal employment opportunity policy,
- the formal internal and external dissemination of the policy,
- the establishment of responsibilities for implementation of the programme,
- the identification of problem areas,
- the setting of goals and objectives to correct these problems,
- the development and execution of action-oriented programmes to eliminate problems and promote the meeting of goals and timetables,
- the design and implementation of an internal audit to measure effectiveness,
- the active support of local and national community action programmes designed to improve the employment opportunities of minorities and women,
- consideration of minorities and women currently in the workforce having the requisite skills who might be recruited through an affirmative action programme.

Each of these components is then further elaborated in the regulations. We need expand on only one. Hidden away in these items is one which, in the British context, would be at the core of an affirmative action plan. It consists of that set of steps that should be taken to increase the pool of available and qualified minorities from which suitable job candidates can be chosen. In short, they are steps to increase the number of minorities in the interview room. The theory of affirmative action (but not of preferential treatment) is then that merit and merit alone must count. Affirmative action stops before selection takes place (again, in theory).

The affirmative steps suggested in the regulations are the following (it is not intended to be an exhaustive list):

- detailed examinations of all job descriptions to ensure that they accurately reflect job functions and are consistent between different facilities;
- the validation of all worker-specifications and required qualifications to ensure they are not indirectly discriminatory,[12] and where they do have disparate impact and are to be retained, that they are justified by 'business necessity';[13]
- approved position descriptions and worker specifications to be available to all personnel involved in recruiting and selection;
- the entire selection process to be evaluated to ensure freedom from bias;
- careful selection and training of all personnel involved in recruitment, selection, promotion and related practices;
- all selection should conform to the requirements of the EEOC/ OFCCP Uniform Guidelines on Employee Selection Procedures;
- selection techniques other than tests such as informal interviews or applications, the use of arrest records, credit checks and consideration of marital status may also be indirectly discriminatory and should be abandoned if possible;
- recruiting sources must be made as wide as possible to include local, community and national organisations with an interest in promoting employment opportunities for minorities and women;
- steps to be taken to inform such organisations of the work of the company, the types of jobs undertaken and of recruitment plans;
- preparedness to accept applicant referrals from such agencies and from current minority and female staff (a procedure that does not appear to differ in any significant manner from word-of-mouth recruiting which in other circumstances is discouraged);
- special efforts to include minorities and women among personnel staff;
- minority employees to be made available to participate in career days, youth motivation programmes and related activities;
- active participation in 'job fairs';
- active recruitment in secondary schools, junior colleges and colleges with predominant minority enrolments;
- all school recruitment to include special efforts to reach minority students;

- a variety of training schemes in predominantly minority schools and colleges;
- minorities and women to be evident in all recruitment materials;
- use of the minority media for job advertisements;
- equal opportunity for promotion must be ensured.

This extensive list coincides with what in Britain would be called 'affirmative action'. In the United States such action is more explicitly a part of a broader strategy – the overall affirmative action programme. The substance of the list, however, does not differ in any marked degree from the sorts of activities that are promoted in Britain as affirmative action.

It is necessary to elaborate on two other items in the list of affirmative actions to be pursued in fulfilment of an affirmative action programme. These are disparate impact analysis and test validations.

Disparate impact analysis and test validation

A disparate impact analysis may be carried out by an employer as part of his affirmative action programme or by an equal opportunity special-ist from the OFCCP as part of a compliance review. The former is by far the more common and the assessment of tests of all kinds for disparate impact between racial and ethnic groups is now 'big business' in the United States.

The legal recognition of disparate impact as a form of discrimination stems, as we have already seen, from the Supreme Court decisions in *Griggs v. Duke Power.* Disparate impact means in essence that a facially neutral test (or practice), such as a general intelligence test or a general ability test or even a test of manual dexterity, may be passed at different rates by different ethnic or racial groups (or average attainment may be different for different groups). What appears therefore to be a neutral test turns out in practice to have a discriminatory effect and may disbar more members of one group from employment (to the extent that the test is used as a qualifier for hiring). This, of course, may be a necessary if unfortunate consequence if the test is one that measures abilities that are essential for the job. If a test is necessary to establish whether someone has the abilities to be an airline pilot then any discriminatory effects it may have cannot be a major consideration. But not all tests are essential for assessing and predicting critical job performance (see Sher 1987) and if they are not, and have a disparate impact, then they *unnecessarily* discriminate and ought to be aban-doned. Apart from job performance prediction, however, there is one other ground on which a test that shows disparate impact may be retained (provided that no alternative non-discriminatory test can be found) and that is if it can be shown to be justified on grounds of 'business necessity'. A disparate impact analysis, therefore, will usually go hand in hand with the validation of a test for predictive performance and/or business necessity. Because they have historically held, and continue to hold, focal positions in the affirmative action process, we shall devote some space here to an examination of disparate impact analysis and test validation and some of the arguments that have developed around them and also review the rise and (partial) fall of 'race-norming' of test scores which is itself a development out of disparate impact theory.

Four years were to elapse after *Griggs* before the Supreme Court tackled the details of establishing the disparate impact of tests. The issue arose in *Albermarle Paper Co. v. Moody* (1975) (which we have already cited in the context of 'make-whole' relief) and centred around how to establish a sufficient showing of job-relatedness of an aptitude test that had disparate impact (that is, to validate it because of its capacity to predict job performance). The Albermarle Paper Co. had in fact conducted validation exercises on its tests but the Court found these and the tests' predictive performance substantially lacking. In the body of its findings (which we need not detail here), the Court for the first time established some of the ground-rules for measuring disparate impact and conducting validation. The following year, validation was again put to the test by the Supreme Court in *Washington v. Davis* (1976). In this case, the Court found a test not to be unlawful (and in effect validated it), even though it had a very significant disparate impact, on the grounds that it was a valuable predictor of performance not on a job *per se* but on a training programme. The performance correlation between the training programme and the job itself (as police officers) had not been established. The message sent by the Court to proponents of the disparate impact theory seemed less than encouraging but again at least some of the post-*Griggs* ground-rules on validation had been established. There was a cumulative message, however, from these and other, lower court findings – and that was that establishing disparate impact and validating tests on the grounds of job-relatedness was a serious business and was to be taken seriously. So seriously in fact that many companies, faced with what they saw to be a nightmare of statistical complexity and financial cost, abandoned the use of scored tests altogether. (Unscored tests and procedures – such as interviews – are, if anything, more difficult to absolve from disparate impact and to validate but they are less complex and offer more room for manoeuvre.)

For most companies however – and especially federal contractors – there was little alternative to subjecting all ability and aptitude tests that they used to disparate impact analysis and, if disparate impact were established, to abandoning the tests and looking for others that suited requirements but were not discriminatory, or validating their existing tests by establishing job performance relevance or relation to business necessity. The Uniform Guidelines on Employee Selection Procedures stipulate that:

> The use of any selection procedure which has an adverse impact on the hiring, promotion or other employment or membership oppor- tunities of members of any race, sex or ethnic group, will be considered to be discriminatory and inconsistent with these guide- lines, unless the procedure has been validated in accordance with these guidelines.
>
> (United States Code of Federal Regulations 1989: 41 CFR 60–3.3(A))

Conforming with this requirement was (and is), as Anthony and Bowen point out, an expensive business (see Anthony and Bowen 1977: 616–17). The elements of a disparate impact analysis, whether carried out by a company or by OFCCP as part of a compliance review, are as follows. The first step is to establish that such tests and procedures as are in place are uniformly applied – that is, applied, measured, interpreted and used in the same manner for all groups. Evidence of non-uniform use between minority groups and between them and the majority group would constitute a prima-facie case of disparate *treatment* – or intentional discrimination. Second, the test or procedure must be established as being facially neutral – that is, that it appears not to have regard to race, sex or any other prohibited factor. A job description that required being white as a condition would not be facially neutral and would again constitute disparate treatment (and disparate impact analysis would be irrelevant). The third step is the crucial one in the analysis and consists of establishing the degree of disparate impact of a test or procedure (if any). To be discriminatory, a test must show 'substantial impact' – that is, there must be a substantial disparity between the numbers of protected and unprotected group members the test 'rejects'. 'Substantial impact' is then interpreted as being statistically significant at a level of two or more standard deviations, though the more commonly known measure is the 'four-fifths rule' which is in effect an initial screen. For discrimination to be established statistical significance must be shown. The four-fifths rule is articulated in the Code of Federal Regulations thus:

> A selection rate for any race, sex, or ethnic group, which is less than four fifths (or eighty *per cent*) of the rate for the group with the highest rate will generally be regarded by Federal enforcement agencies as evidence of adverse impact . . .
>
> (United States Code of Federal Regulations 1989: 41 CFR 60–3.4(D))

In more specific terms, if less than 80 per cent of (say) African- Americans taking a test pass at the level achieved by all members of the group that scores highest, the test is deemed to have adverse (or disparate) impact and to be discriminatory. Its continued use without validation would then leave an employer open to a charge of unintentional discrimination under Title VII following the Griggs Doctrine.

Having established disparate impact, therefore, the test must be abandoned or validated for job-relatedness or business necessity. Thus, as we have noted, if the test is an effective and necessary predictor of job performance and no other test exists with similar predictive powers but no, or less, disparate impact, then it may be retained despite its discriminatory effect. Alternatively (and until *Ward's Cove*), if the employer could show that the test was necessary for the safe and efficient running of the business, then, again, it could be retained. An obvious example would be a language test in English comprehension that had an adverse impact on Hispanics. Such a test might pass the business necessity standard in jobs where fluent conversational English was necessary, but not (for example) in a factory where English was not a requirement for the job and all necessary instructions and safety notices could be posted in translation.

The Supreme Court finding in *Ward's Cove v. Atonio* was, as we have noted earlier, a key factor in subsequent attempts to get a new Civil Rights Act passed. The weakening of the business necessity standard by the Court in that case was one component of what many saw to be a broader attack on affirmative action. The Court, by a 5–4 majority, allowed the employer's appeal. This is what the majority opinion said about 'business necessity':

> Though we have phrased the query differently in different cases, it is generally well established that at the justification stage of such a disparate impact case, the dispositive issue is whether a challenged practice *serves, in a significant way, the legitimate employment goals of the employer.*
> ... there is no requirement that the challenged practice be 'essential' or 'indispensable' to the employer's business for it to pass muster: this degree of scrutiny would be almost impossible for most employers to meet . . .
> (*Ward's Cove Packing Co. v. Atonio* as quoted in *United States Law Week* 1989: 57 LW 4588, emphasis added)

Business necessity was no longer to be the standard to be met in order to use a test showing disparate impact. The Court chose to interpret this as meaning 'essential' and 'indispensable' which it then claimed was an unreachable standard. The standard had to be weaker otherwise too many valuably diagnostic tests would be invalidated. And this new standard was to be in service of 'the legitimate employment goals of the employer' which, as Justice White pointed out, was more in conformity with the standard required in disparate treatment cases (see Murphy 1989: 2). It hardly needs saying, however, that 'the legitimate employment goals' of an employer is a phrase open to a wide variety of interpretations and has the potential for permitting the use of far more tests having disparate impact. The status quo ante *Ward's Cove*, however, has been partially restored with the passing of the 1991 Civil Rights Act, as we shall see later.

Even though the design and production of culturally neutral tests having no disparate impact has become a major business in the human relations field in the United States, there is still dispute about whether a truly culturally neutral test exists. The debate is too technically complex to warrant examination here but there is evidence that the ways in which cultural bias might enter tests and their administration, scoring and interpretation are so multi-factorial that pure neutrality is a chimera (see for example Flaugher, 1977). Again, Pearn, after a review of mainly American research, concluded that 'there is no such thing as a culture-fair test' (Pearn 1978). Whether or not these cautions are true, it does seem almost certainly to be the case that the search for *more* neutrality (less disparate impact) has led to a reduction in diagnostic and predictive capacity in the field of employment testing. So also has the abandonment of tests that are predictive but have disparate impact and could not reach the 'business necessity' standard. For many jobs, this might not matter if the benefits to be gained from what must always be a fairly approximate science of performance prediction are marginal. Put simply, it doesn't much matter how you choose employees for many lower-skilled jobs and the use of expensive tests and their validation will not reap any measurable increases in efficiency or output. At higher skill levels and for many professional jobs, it will matter more and there can be little doubt that a price has been paid for trading off predictive performance for less disparate impact. Affirmative action therefore is not, and has not been, costless, as some may like to argue. The costs have been financial, moral and, in this case, in efficiency and possibly in economic terms. Whether the price is worth paying we leave for detailed assessment later.

Before we leave the subject of testing and disparate impact, we must consider another and more contentious aspect – what has become known technically as 'within-group scoring' but more commonly as 'race-norming'. The essence of this procedure is that is converts raw scores on a test into percentiles *within* each ethnic or racial group. Thus, the score of a black candidate is compared only with those of other blacks and not with all other candidates. Results are then reported not as a score but as within a percentile range. A raw score that would put a candidate within a certain percentile for whites (or for all candidates) will put the candidate into a much higher percentile on the within-black (or within-Hispanic) ranking. Only the latter within-group ranking is then used.

The most extensive use of race-norming has been made by the US government itself in the form of the Employment Service of the Labor

Department. In 1981 the Labor Department encouraged state employment services to use its General Aptitude Test Battery (GATB) for screening candidates for jobs in state agencies and the private sector. At the same time, it encouraged within-group scoring on the GATB (see Blits and Gottfredson 1990a: 20, 1990b: 4).[14] The report that an employer would then receive from the employment agency on a candidate would include the candidate's performance on the GATB but *only* as a within-group percentile. The effect of this is to abandon any pretence that all candidates of whatever race are being compared equally. But the employer might not be aware of this, or, if she were, would have no way of comparing candidates of different races. Whatever else race-norming does, it changes the rules of the merit system.

In 1986 the Justice Department ordered the Labor Department to cease promoting race-norming on the grounds that it was in violation of Title VII. The Labor Department agreed not to *expand* its promotion of race-norming until a review of its effects in relation to GATB by the National Research Council (a branch of the National Academy of Sciences) was completed. The review appeared in 1989, concluded that the GATB disadvantaged blacks and Hispanics and recommended that it continued to be race-normed for these two groups (Hartigan and Wigdor 1989). At this stage, race-norming entered the battle for a new Civil Rights Act (*Congressional Quarterly Researcher* 1991a: 289). It was probably one of the least easily defended components of affirmative action in the long series of trade-offs that finally produced the Act and was made unlawful in the following amendment to the Civil Rights Act 1964 (in effect, a new subsection to section 703 of that Act):

> It shall be an unlawful employment practice for a respondent . . . to adjust the scores of, use different cutoff scores for, or otherwise alter the results of, employment related tests on the basis of race, color, religion, sex, or national origin.
>
> (Civil Rights Act 1991: s. 106)

Standards of compliance

Where a contractor has established under-utilisation and set goals to rectify this, the goal for any particular job type will normally be the availability rate for minorities and timetables will be established to meet this goal by means of positive actions over a year or more (though there must be annual interim goals if the timetable is longer than one year). The essence of the programme is that it is 'do-able' and realistically achievable, and the affirmative actions that are taken (such as outreach) must be tailored to produce the desired results. And the OFCCP will require evidence that appropriate action is being taken in compliance with the programme. The standard for measuring compliance, however, is not the achievement of the goals, but rather a showing that 'good faith efforts' have been made to achieve the goals. Thus, as Cooper has noted:

> Simply, good faith efforts comprise the standard of compliance with Executive Order 11246. A contractor who can demonstrate good faith efforts is in compliance . . . no matter how far the contractor is from fulfilling his established goals in the affirmative action program.
>
> (Cooper 1987: 5.2)

The contractor is best able to show good faith efforts by demonstrating that he has taken a range of affirmative actions which are tailored to his particular situation and that he has, in effect, done all that could reasonably be expected in pursuit of the goals.

Now this aspect of goal measurement is often cited as being what distinguishes a goal from a quota. A goal is just that – something to aim for but not necessarily meet – whilst a quota must be met, and when met, not exceeded. The distinction is rather more hazy than this implies, however. Notwithstanding that good faith efforts are the measure of compliance there is often the pressure for a variety of reasons to go to considerable lengths to meet the goal – as if it were a quota. One relatively common practice (which the OFCCP now tries to discourage) is the 'recycling' or 'pirating' of minorities – that is, enticing minority group employees away from another company when there is no possibility of increasing their employment from the availability pool. This type of activity is symptomatic of what might be called the 'culture of affirmative action', as we shall demonstrate in the next chapter. Before that, however, we must introduce the most recent legislation and the circumstances that produced it.

THE REHNQUIST COURT AND THE CIVIL RIGHTS ACT 1991

Between 1986 and 1991 the Supreme Court made nine rulings which in varying degrees narrowed the reach of anti-discrimination law and practice including affirmative action. In the 1988/89 term alone under Chief Justice Rehnquist there were seven rulings which attempted to rein in anti-discrimination and affirmative action practice. The Court's actions were seen by civil rights proponents as quite deliberate and purposeful. They were not just a coincidence of cases. Here was the Supreme Court trying to rewrite civil rights law and practice to fit its own conservative mould. Not only did the 1989 rulings appear to undermine parts of the 1984 Civil Rights Act, they also seemed to many observers to reverse the Griggs Doctrine which, as we have seen, underpinned much equal opportunity and affirmative action practice (see Edwards 1991). There was a civil rights backlash and an immediate attempt to reinstate what the Supreme Court had struck down, in the form of a new Civil Rights Bill designed to close the loopholes opened up by the Court. This was vetoed by President Bush and re-introduced in 1991 with amendments. The administration introduced its own bill the same year and a hybrid version of the two was passed in October.

The 1989 rulings

For present purposes we need only summarise the key aspects of the seven 1989 rulings. Some will be the subject of further discussion in subsequent chapters.

Of *City of Richmond v. J.A. Croson Company* (1989) and *Ward's Cove Packing v. Atonio* (1989) there will be much more to say later. At issue in *Richmond* was a city set-aside programme in which 30 per cent of the dollar value of all construction work should go to minority businesses. The plan was struck down on the grounds that the city had failed to demonstrate 'identified discrimination' and that the programme did not constitute a properly tailored remedy. In short, the Court wanted much more precise evidence of discrimination and an affirmative action programme that was tailored to correct the *identified* wrongdoing. (What this entailed, among other things, was that any remedial efforts be limited to the particular minority group that had been harmed – in this case, African-Americans – and not, as had been the case with Richmond's set-aside programme, open to any and all minority groups.) This stemmed from the decision of the Court to judge the Richmond case as a constitutional one and to apply 'strict scrutiny' under the equal protection clause. This required that the city showed a 'compelling interest' why a race-based programme should be implemented. Six of the nine judges decided that Richmond had failed to show any such compelling public interest (see Murphy 1989, Lively 1992: Chapter 6).

The finding in *Ward's Cove* had more far reaching consequences than any of the other six 1989 cases. We have touched on it earlier but it is worth reminding ourselves of its key features. In essence, *Ward's Cove* shifted the burden of proof of discrimination from the employer to the employees; it required that precise and particular discriminatory practices be identified (rather than statistical disparate impact) and it made employer-justification of disparate impact practices much easier by abandoning the 'business necessity' requirement and substituting the much looser 'serving legitimate employer goals'. All this made it much more difficult for employees to demonstrate discrimination and in particular appeared to negate the Griggs Doctrine which, as we have already noted, was so fundamental to anti-discrimination and affirmative action practice (see Murphy 1989, Bowser 1990: 5).

In *Martin v. Wilks* (1989) the Supreme Court opened the way for retrospective challenges to consent decrees that included agreed goals for minority hiring. A group of white firefighters in Birmingham,

Alabama, was allowed to bring a discrimination suit against a consent decree to which they had not been an original party (even though their representatives had). This was seen as opening the way for endless challenges to consent decrees in every state (*Congressional Quarterly Researcher* 1991a: 288, *Equal Opportunities Review* 1989c: 24).

In *Lorance v. AT&T Technologies* (1989) the Supreme Court imposed a time limit of 300 days within which employees could challenge a seniority plan as discriminatory even though they might not be aware within that time that they had been adversely affected (*Congressional Quarterly Researcher* 1991a: 288).

In another sex discrimination case (*Price Waterhouse v. Hopkins* 1989) the Court found that even if discrimination has been shown, the defendant would not be liable if he or she could demonstrate that they would have come to the same decision even in the absence of any discrimination.

The other two cases are of less importance in the present context. In *Patterson v. McLean Credit Union* (1989) the Court interpreted Title 42 of the US Code as applying only to discrimination in the process of hiring and not once in employ, and *Independent Federation of Flight Attendants v. Zipes* (1989) made it more difficult for parties who prevail in job discrimination suits to win the cost of attorney's fees.

Collectively, these rulings, but in particular the undermining of the Griggs Doctrine, the requirement for programmes to be closely tailored to meet identified discriminatory practices, the shift in burden of proof, the weakening of business necessity and the permissibility of retrospective challenge, constituted a serious curtailment of the reach of affirmative action and the ability to bring, and win, discrimination cases.

There then began two years of continual wrangling over what should, and could, be done to reinstate the damaged parts of the 1964 Act and reverse the trend of the Supreme Court. The first substantive response was the introduction of a new Civil Rights Bill, sponsored by Edward Kennedy in the Senate and Augustus Hawkins in the House. At the same time, the Bush administration, whilst arguing that the Supreme Court rulings did not presage the need for new legislation, announced its own more limited measure designed to counter the *Lorance* and *Patterson* rulings.

The Kennedy/Hawkins bill succeeded in getting a majority but fell short by one vote of the two-thirds majority required to overcome the inevitable presidential veto. It was, claimed President Bush, a 'quota bill' and would force employers into setting quotas as an insurance against discrimination charges. The following year the Democrats reintroduced a Civil Rights Bill (HR 1) but this time shorn of any language that might suggest quotas and with an explicit disclaimer that it either permitted or required the setting of quotas. President Bush said it was still a 'quotas bill' and announced that the administration would introduce its own bill but one with a much wider sweep than the one announced the year before.

There followed a period of intensive bargaining during which a compromise bill was hammered out with both parties claiming that the other had had to make greater concessions. It was the administration that was labouring under a handicap, however, because co-terminous with this bargaining were the confirmation hearings for Clarence Thomas, the President's nominee to the Supreme Court, during which Thomas was accused of sexual harassment by Anita Hill, his one-time subordinate at the EEOC. Wherever the truth lay it was a deep embarrassment to the administration to have confirmation hearings for a Supreme Court judge hijacked by petty and detailed sexual accusations and rebuttals.

A compromise bill was eventually put together – one that would command a majority and win the assent of the President, but only at the expense of some important ambiguities that it was left to the courts to thrash out. Nonetheless, it was generally acknowledged that the Civil Rights Act 1991 reversed more Supreme Court rulings than any other piece of legislation for decades.

So apparent were the loopholes and ambiguities in the Act that the legislators agreed to insert a three-paragraph memorandum in the Congressional Record that would constitute the Act's 'exclusive legislative history'. This was in effect an attempt to define key terms and meanings in the Act and limit the scope for courts in future to read lawmakers' intentions into the statements of senators during debate on the Act. Thus, for example, the 'exclusive legislative history', in an attempt to pin down a meaning for 'business necessity' rather than leave it open to the multiplicity of interpretations that might be gleaned from what was said in the Senate, states: 'The terms "business necessity" and "job related" are intended to reflect the concepts of Griggs v. Duke Power (1971) and other Supreme Court decisions prior to Ward's Cove Packing Co. v. Atonio' (*Congressional Quarterly Almanac* 1991: 257).

The Act reversed some, though not all, of the seven 1989 rulings. Most particularly it reinstated the burden of proof in disparate impact cases on the employer but still required the identification by plaintiffs of particular discriminatory practices except where this was impossible. As a reversal of *Patterson*, the Act bars racial bias and harassment during employment as well as at hiring and in response to *Martin v. Wilks* it spelled out rules under which third parties could challenge a consent degree. The rulings in *Price Waterhouse* and *Lorance* were similarly overturned by the Act. *Richmond*, however, because it revolved around the constitutional question of 'strict scrutiny', was not directly addressed by the Act and, in the attempt to reach a compromise bill, neither side, it would seem, wanted to raise that particular hare. In addition to these reversals of specific rulings, the Act made provision for monetary damages, both compensatory and punitive, but at the same time fixed (fairly modest) upper limits.

Two further components of the Act are worth pointing up. The first we have noted earlier in the chapter – that the outlawing of test score 'race-norming' had to be one of the concessions made by the proponents of civil rights. The other was the relatively uncontentious notion of a 'Glass Ceiling Commission', the job of which was to investigate ways of promoting women and minorities from middle management jobs, where their numbers were increasing, into senior management and other decision-making positions, where they remained scarce.

6 Race-conscious practice
The United States

Although affirmative action practice has been widespread in the United States for more than a quarter of a century, and though in many respects it has 'bedded-down' to become normal practice, it continues to raise contentious questions (as well as hackles). Some of these – such as when does affirmative action become preferential treatment; when are quotas permissible; what is so good about the 'merit principle' that it should never be overridden; what is the relationship between seniority rules and the protection of affirmative action gains – seem never to go away and on occasion break out in a new round of controversy (some of it heated and unpleasant) such as that which occurred at Georgetown University Law Center in Washington D.C. in April 1991. No matter how strenuously the official prohibition on preferential treatment is promulgated, there remains a widespread belief that it is commonly practised. That belief is not an unrealistic one as it turns out. Preferential treatment became an issue in the Senate elections in 1990: Senator Jesse Helms of North Carolina ran effective television advertising showing a pair of white hands crumpling up a job rejection slip with a voice-over saying it was a pity, he was the best qualified, but the job had to go to a minority under a racial quota. It neatly encapsulated the fears and resentments of many whites (and especially white working-class males). There was, in the wake of this and other events, such as the good showing in the 1990 elections of David Duke, a former Klansman who made quotas a central plank on his platform, a widespread fear that the debate about race-conscious practice would turn nasty during the presidential election. In the event – and much to the surprise of those concerned with racial issues – neither race in general, nor the quota issue in particular, played any significant part.

This chapter attempts to provide some of the 'feel' of affirmative action practice in the United States and in particular to examine how contentious matters like quotas and preferential treatment are dealt with in practice. We shall then, in a subsequent chapter, examine these questions from a moral and juridical point of view.

As with the studies of private companies and public agencies in Great

Britain, the material that follows is intended only to be illustrative. There is no pretence at representativeness and the material does not constitute systematic or detailed descriptions and analyses of any agency's affirmative action programmes or race-conscious policies.

Four 'agencies' were selected, mainly on the basis of proximity and ease of access. All four are located in the same state but for consistency with the British examples, they are not here identified by name. Two are public agencies – a city administration and a state administration; one is a relatively large state university; and the fourth a large multi-national chemical corporation with headquarters in the same state. The main problems and issues that exercise each of these agencies in the field of race-conscious policy are not all the same, but in addition to identifying the particular concerns of each agency we shall pursue several themes common to all. Among these will be those topics that we have already noted as being of most general concern – the relation between affirmative action and preferential treatment, the use of quotas, overriding merit and the question of redefining qualifications.

CITY OF W

The City of W has a population of just over 70,000, of which at the 1990 census 39.6 per cent were white, 51.6 per cent black, 6.7 per cent of Hispanic origin, 0.4 per cent Asian-Americans, with the small remainder being American Indian or 'other'. It is a relatively poor town; one in ten of the population live in subsidised housing, 16,000 receive food stamps, and 10,000 receive aid to households with dependent children (City of W 1990b). This high poverty rate has not been ameliorated by the influx of financial institutions to the city following on new state Incorporation Laws which make it a very attractive location for large companies. Indeed, the immigration of numbers of young professional people has boosted the price of housing and along with the liberal use of Urban Development Action Grants has created extensive gentrification of property, to the housing detriment of the poor and in particular blacks and Hispanics. Within this context minority employment (and self-employment) are crucial factors in boosting and maintaining the standing of minority communities in the city.

We shall look at two separate components of affirmative action and equal opportunity practice in W. The first is the affirmative action plan of the city itself, and the second the hiring practices of the Public Safety Department in respect of the police force, the latter being illustrative of a robust attitude to affirmative action practice.

City of W workforce

The City of W had a workforce of 1300 in 1990 – a figure that had been growing slowly over the previous few years. In 1988 the workforce stood at 1269, of which 49.6 per cent were white, 44.8 per cent black, 4.9 per cent Hispanic, 0.7 per cent Asian-American and 0.08 per cent American Indian. These ethnic representations compare with figures for the city's labour draw area (which because of a residence qualification for employment is co-terminous with the city boundary) of 39.6 per cent white, 51.6 per cent black, 6.7 per cent Hispanic, with other groups making up the residuum. The ethnic and racial composition of the workforce by job categories for the years 1984 and 1988 are shown in Table 6.1. Despite some notable improvements over the four-year period, particularly in the professional grade, it is clear that blacks remain under-represented (as compared with their representation in the total workforce) in the top four grades and over-represented in the lowest grades.

The plan

The W administration was fully aware of the degree of under-representation (it could hardly not have been, given its obligation to make regular EEO-4 monitoring returns to the EEOC) and was taking action to correct it. But not, it seems, aggressive action. Thus, *The City of W Affirmative Action Plan* (City of W 1990b) bears more resemblance to a policy statement than to a plan as such. It does not contain data on the ethnic and racial composition of the workforce, nor any target figures for the future. It does contain details of good practice (including outreach to schools and colleges) but these are not linked to any plan or strategy for attaining goals. Neither is there any timetable by which actions should be achieved. This want of a structured plan of action, however, is to some extent offset by the fact that the organisation is a relatively small one and much can be (and was) achieved by informal contacts between the Department of Personnel and other departments.

The aims of affirmative action procedures are encapsulated in the equal employment opportunity statement issued over the signature of the mayor of W which concludes: 'Our ultimate goal is representation at all levels of responsibility which approximates the composition of the community we serve, for it is to these citizens we must answer' (City of W 1990c). A gloss was added to this, however, by the Affirmative Action Officer, who confirmed that while representativeness (or representation throughout the workforce proportional to that in the population of the city) was the broad aim of the city's policy, reducing the difference in the two distributions was a goal that was being worked to 'in an informal way'. This latter point was by way of emphasising that they were working to a goal and not a quota. And in practice this was true for almost all departments insofar as their affirmative action measures were not aggressively pursued and stopped short of any preferential treatment.

Table 6.1 Ethnic/racial composition of City of W workforce by EEO-4 job category, 1988 and 1984

Ethnic/racial composition 1988

EEO-4 job category	White		Black		Hispanic		Asian-American		American Indian		Total	
	No.	%	No.	%	No.	%	No.	%	No.	%	No.	%
Official/admin.	44	72.1	15	24.6	1	1.6	1	1.6	0	0	61	100
Professionals	105	62.9	57	34.1	2	1.2	3	1.8	0	0	167	100
Technicians	88	68.2	36	27.9	3	2.3	2	1.6	0	0	129	100
Protective services	220	56.8	143	36.9	23	5.9	1	0.3	1	1.5	387	100
Para-professionals	35	53.0	27	40.9	2	3.0	1	1.5	0	0	66	100
Office/clerical	38	30.6	78	62.9	8	6.5	0	0	0	0	124	100
Skilled craft	66	45.2	74	50.7	6	4.1	0	0	0	0	146	100
Service/maintenance	33	17.5	138	73.0	17	9.0	1	0.5	0	0	189	100
Total	629	49.6	568	44.8	62	4.9	9	0.7	1	0.08	1269	100

Ethnic/racial composition 1984

EEO-4 job category	White		Black		Hispanic		Asian-American		American Indian		Total	
	No.	%	No.	%	No.	%	No.	%	No.	%	No.	%
Official/admin	19	76.0	5	20.0	0	0	1	4.0	0	0	25	100
Professionals	122	74.8	36	22.1	3	1.8	2	1.2	0	0	163	100
Technicians	95	73.1	29	22.3	4	3.1	2	1.5	0	0	130	100
Protective services	232	60.7	131	34.3	18	4.7	1	0.3	0	0	382	100
Para-professionals	41	58.6	26	37.1	2	2.8	1	1.4	0	0	70	100
Office/clerical	54	43.2	68	54.4	3	2.4	0	0	0	0	125	100
Skilled craft	73	45.9	82	51.6	3	1.9	1	0.6	0	0	159	100
Service/maintenance	29	15.6	148	79.6	9	4.8	0	0	0	0	186	100
Total	665	53.6	525	42.3	42	3.4	8	0.6	0	0	1240	100
City of W	–	39.6	–	51.6	–	6.7	–	0.4	–	0.09	–	100

Source: City of W (1990a)

Affirmative action practice

Affirmative action in W is seen as essentially the removal of barriers to equality of opportunity and the use of outreach measures to encourage more minority job applicants. Outreach practices are not designed solely or even mainly to attract minority applicants for particular job openings but rather to promote the city administration in general as a valuable source of employment for minorities. In pursuit of this latter element, the Department of Personnel and the Affirmative Action Office encourage the local media to include minority employees in their coverage of the administration, promote occupation training programmes, provide work opportunity and experience for minority youth, continually emphasise the affirmative action policy of the administration to all local community and voluntary groups, and maintain personal contact with local schools and colleges with high minority enrolments. Broadly similar methods are used when attempting to attract minority candidates for particular job vacancies but with more emphasis – as would be expected – in targeting job advertisements and using special recruiting materials, including Spanish translations.

The candidate selection process is subjected to scrutiny under the affirmative action programme to ensure that all the criteria and techniques used to screen candidates are 'fair and non-discriminatory'. Not surprisingly, in the light of our earlier discussion of adverse impact, a great deal of effort is put into ensuring that no adverse impact is shown by any tests and procedures used and that where there is adverse impact, it can, if necessary, be justified by job-relatedness. A similar scrutiny is applied to all tests and procedures used for the purposes of promotion and transfer.

At the point of selection – for hiring or promotion – there is a strong injunction to use merit and merit alone as the criterion (though as we shall see below, 'merit' has a flexible meaning). The Affirmative Action Officer acknowledged that many other agencies and companies did use preferential treatment – if not quotas – but emphasised that it just was not possible in W if only because the trade unions would not accept it. Furthermore, at least until the interview stage, the hiring department would not know the race or ethnicity of applicants because this is entered by the candidate on a tear-off slip on the application form which is removed by the Department of Personnel before the forms are sent to departments. (Many Hispanic people, of course, would remain identifiable by the name on the form.) There is, however, one small qualification to this overt policy of no preferential treatment which is that in a tie-break between two equally qualified and suitable candidates, one of whom is white and the other minority, the minority candidate would be chosen.

Merit

We have noted that in hiring and promotion procedures the city administration will, at the point of selection, use only merit. That is stated in unequivocal terms in the *Affirmative Action Plan* (City of W 1990d) and was reaffirmed by the Affirmative Action Officer. Merit can mean many things, however, and in W it means more than qualifications. It was acknowledged that it was no bad thing to consider a candidate's 'suitability' or 'compatibility' for a job or position. Many measurement tests, it was argued, are arbitrary (in terms of performance prediction) and difficult to interpret. Small numerical differences in scores could not be used to distinguish between candidates. There was good reason, therefore, to use a wider range of diagnostic measures including assessments of productivity and efficiency (not only *of* the candidate but also of the effect of the candidate *on* these factors within a unit or department), and 'profile modelling' to assess how a candidate might fit a job and a position within a department. The use of such a variety of measures, it was argued, introduced a greater degree of flexibility into the selection process which, overall, could increase the chances of a minority candidate being selected. We shall consider the 'merit' principle in greater depth in a later chapter.

The pool

The single greatest constraint upon the employment of more black and Hispanic people in the city administration, according to the Affirmative Action Officer, was non-availability. One part of this problem consisted of the 'residence qualification' used by the city whereby all employees of the administration must live within the city boundaries. And, given the high cost of housing in the city which we noted earlier, few people who might want to work for W want to live there (and particularly since many senior administrative positions may turn over every four years with changes in the political administration). The effective minority availability, therefore, is confined to the city itself. There is little chance of attracting minorities from outside. Within the city availability is restricted by the shortage of qualified minorities which thus far, outreach training programmes have done little to improve. In consequence, it is easier to employ (and achieve utilisation of) relatively low-skilled minority employees and much more difficult to increase representation at higher administrative and managerial levels.

The City of W is not unique in this (though it is trammelled by its residence qualification); it will turn out that an inadequate pool of qualified minorities is the single greatest limitation to increasing minority representation in those positions where they are most under-utilised.

Notwithstanding this limitation to increasing the numbers of minorities in higher graded jobs, some progress has been made by the City of W as the data in Table 6.1 indicate. During the short period covered by these figures, the proportion of officials and administrators who were black increased from 20.0 per cent to 24.6 per cent and for professionals the increase was far more impressive – from 22.1 per cent to 34.1 per cent. At the other end of the scale, the over-representation of blacks in low- and semi-skilled jobs declined from 79.6 per cent (compared with black representation in the workforce as a whole of 42.3 per cent) to 73.0 per cent in 1988 (against a total workforce representation of 44.8 per cent). Over the same period the number of Hispanic employees increased by twenty (and from 3.4 per cent to 4.9 per cent of the workforce) but most of this gain was in the lower job grades. The Deputy Personnel Director admitted that these gains could not with certainty be attributed to affirmative action efforts entirely, but he was certain that affirmative action was largely responsible.

Despite the relatively modest affirmative action efforts of the city, therefore (at least compared with the aggressive approach of some universities and private sector establishments), the gains in minority employment, at least for blacks, have been quite significant as judged over the short time span of 1984–88.

The W police force

The Department of Police, along with the Department of Fire, falls under the Office of Public Safety which manages its own personnel functions (that is, independently of the W Department of Personnel). This independence provides the potential for greater flexibility in effecting affirmative action for minorities. It is a potential that has been exploited by a dynamic Director of Public Safety with forthright views of the kind of police force he wants. Whilst there is no policy of preferring minorities in recruitment and promotion (indeed, as elsewhere in W, there is a formal policy of non-preference), the Director has used whatever flexibility exists in the personnel system to enhance minority representation. Progress is being made but it is 'an uphill struggle', and as Table 6.2 shows, there remains a very marked imbalance. Whether the figures for W City are taken as an approximate draw area or as representative of the make-up of the community to be policed, they show a very different ethnic pattern from that of the police force at every rank – including new recruits.

Equal opportunity policy

There is no written recruitment and promotion policy for the police force other than the general W policy statement we have already

Table 6.2 Ethnic/racial composition of W police force by rank, 1990

Rank	Ethnic/racial group					
	White %	Black %	Hispanic %	Other %	Total No.	%
Chief of Police	100.0	0	0	0	1	100
Inspector	66.7	33.3	0	0	3	100
Captain	85.7	14.3	0	0	7	100
Lieutenant	69.2	23.1	7.7	0	13	100
Sergeant	81.2	16.7	2.1	0	48	100
Patrol Officer	62.7	30.8	5.3	1.2	169	100
Recruits	65.5	31.0	3.4	0	29	100
Total	67.4	27.4	4.4	0.7	270	100
W City draw area[a]	39.6	51.6	6.7	2.1	–	100

Source: City of W Office of Public Safety (1990)
Note: [a] In practice, recruitment extends beyond the city boundary.

described. The guiding principle for the desired composition of the police force, adopted in 1980, is the same as for the city administration as a whole – that is, proportionality. The ethnic and racial composition of the force ought to reflect that of the community it serves. For the Director of Public Safety, however, this was as much a matter of consequence as of justice or equality of opportunity. Only by having an ethnic mix that reflected that of the city, he argued, would it be possible for police officers to have a sensitivity to and understanding of people's problems and anxieties. Otherwise, there was the danger – all too apparent in some other cities – of the police looking like an 'occupying force'. A better ethnic mix, he said, was at the core of producing a less confrontational police force, less crime and a safer city while at the same time creating good relationships between the police and the communities. The current policy, therefore, is that entrance classes to the police should reflect the demographics of the city and should therefore contain at least 50 per cent minorities (at which level there would still be under-representation).

Outreach

It is not possible even nearly to approach a 50 per cent minority entrance class by confining recruitment to the city itself. The first thing that must happen is that the 'residence qualification' rule must be overridden, and the Department of Safety now targets and attempts to recruit from colleges with high black enrolments and from traditional black colleges as far away as Philadelphia and New Jersey (up to 100 miles away). This particular form of outreach is driven by a decision made in 1984 that recruits must have *at least* a High School Diploma or the General Equivalence Diploma but that college experience would be preferred; hence the drive to get black college graduates.

In the four years to 1990 between five and ten black college recruits were taken on per year by this means, but though they are good recruits, it is not a cost-effective way of hiring minorities. Reaching out to colleges at distances of 50–100 miles is expensive both in time and finances. It is a policy that will be continued nonetheless because there are few alternatives: quite simply, it is very hard to find blacks who qualify and who want to be policemen: 'If they are good, they will go to higher paid jobs in "SA"' (the large multinational chemical corporation based in W and the subject of a subsequent part of this chapter). The image of the police in W is, however, improving and is increasingly seen as a good profession for both black men and women to enter. Whether or not this will continue to be the case, however, may depend on potential recruitees' perceptions of how blacks currently in the police force progress up the ladder. Optimism may turn sour if too many are kept from senior positions by the 'glass ceiling'.

The Director of Public Safety is black and he has put much effort into attracting high quality black recruits. The recruitment of Hispanics, however (6.7 per cent of the population of W), he acknowledges is a more difficult task. There is no obvious recruitment source comparable to black colleges (other colleges with high Hispanic enrolment are targeted) and the psychological barriers to enrolment are as great, and possibly greater, than for blacks.

Recruitment procedures

The Director of Public Safety has taken the view that an exploitation of the flexibility that exists in the recruitment procedures provides the best opportunity to increase minority representation. The procedure for entry to the uniformed ('sworn') force follows these steps:

- application,
- interview,
- 'pencil and paper' test,
- physical test (endurance),
- criminal history check,
- background check (including interviews with people from the candidate's neighbourhood),
- Interview Board (with second-level officers),
- placed on list for interview with Chief of Police,
- test by psychologist.

A candidate can fail at any point in this procedure and failure precludes progress to the next stage. All the tests involved have been analysed for adverse impact for both black and Hispanic groups and are continually monitored to detect any new or emerging impact. All tests that have an adverse impact have been validated and only those necessary for job performance have been retained.

Nonetheless, the procedures weed out more blacks as not reaching the required standard (and the failure rate for Hispanics is between that for blacks and whites), and this creates very significant difficulties for a policy of increasing minority representation. In particular, black applicants have higher fail rates on the pencil and paper test and they fail the psychological test at twice the rate for whites.[1] Third, both black and Hispanic candidates have higher failure rates on the criminal history check. (The Director of Public Safety noted that 'a high proportion' of black candidates fail on this test.)

The momentum remains, however, to increase minority representation and this has served to bend some of the constraints in the selection procedures. Within an official policy of 'no preference', therefore, a degree of flexibility has been introduced which enhances the chances of minority applicants being accepted and of being promoted once in the force. It may not in strict terminology constitute preferential treatment, but it is a process of readjusting selection procedures (and the concept of merit) to give every assistance to minority recruitment. And it is common practice – in the public and private sectors and in universities – as will become apparent in the course of this chapter.

First, the original regulation that *any* history of criminal activity debarred entry to the police force has been amended. Now, minor criminal misdemeanours are no longer a barrier to entry. Anything other than minor criminal behaviour however continues to block eligibility. Second, the pass mark of 70 on the written test is now treated as a flexible guide rather than a pass-or-fail mark. Third, black officers are always present at tests and interviews. Fourth, there is always an assumption in favour of a minority candidate at the margins in tests and interviews. Fifth, despite official denials of preference, the presumption in favour of a minority candidate does mean on occasions that, *at the margin*, a less well qualified minority candidate will be appointed over a better qualified (or – significantly – a 'better educated') white applicant. Sixth, 'merit' is seen to consist of a wide variety of components, reaching far beyond performance on tests. There are many qualities required in a policeman, including knowledge of, and sensitivity to, the community he or she will be policing. If that community happens to be predominantly black or Hispanic, then being black or Hispanic may be a component of merit for the job.[2] The qualifier must always be however – as the Director strongly emphasised – that the minority recruits *must* be qualified and the best that can be got. Policing minority communities with incompetent minority police serves no good purpose. (And the same applies to white police in white communities of course.) The argument from 'sensitive policing' appears an attractive one, but when broadened out to a general argument from consequence, its moral ambiguity is exposed. We shall discuss this at greater length in a later chapter. The sixth form of 'bending' occurs in promotion procedures. On the assumption that test batteries lack sufficient precision to justify individual ranking of all potential promotees, they are placed in four bands. Promotion is from band one and all candidates in this band must be promoted before anyone from band two is considered. There are normally more minority candidates in bands three and four than in one and two but the system does enable the promotion of minorities if they can be 'pushed' into the top band and it was argued 'we try to ensure some minorities in the top band'.

There is, in all this, so far as the Director of Public Safety is concerned, an element of compensation: 'The best Affirmative Action Program in the world is friendship. It is what whites have been using for generations. So we are just trying to equalise opportunities.' Progress in changing the ethnic composition of the W police force will be slow for several reasons, among the most important of which are the limited pool of even potentially eligible minorities, the disqualificatory hurdles, the existing imbalance and the cumbersome method of having to bend the rules. The Director of Public Safety was, however, convinced that without pushing the boundaries of affirmative action into preferential treatment, progress towards better representation would be negligible.

STATE OF D

The representation of ethnic and racial minorities in the workforce of the State of D is shown in Table 6.3 along with the composition of the population of the state. (It is worth noting in passing that the proportions of white and non-white population in the state are almost exactly the reverse of those in W City – the state's largest urban centre.) D is a small state however and for employment purposes the labour draw area for the state administration may extend beyond the state boundaries to encompass the Standard Metropolitan Statistical Area.

Taking the state figures as an *approximate guide* only (that is, *not* assuming proportionality is the measure of success nor using state data as availability data), it is evident that whites are somewhat underrepresented and blacks are over-represented in the workforce as a whole. Furthermore, blacks are only plainly under-represented in the top two job categories (and only by 4.5 percentage points for professionals). Blacks do, however, remain heavily over-represented in semi-and unskilled jobs.

Table 6.3 Ethnic/racial composition of the State of D workforce by EEO-4 job category, 1989

EEO-4 job category	*Ethnic/racial composition: 1989 (%)*						
	White	*Black*	*Hispanic*	*Asian- American*	*American Indian*	*Total*	
	%	%	%	%	%	*No.*	%
Official/admin	89.3	8.2	0.2	2.0	0.2	402	100
Professionals	82.3	12.9	1.2	3.5	0.1	2852	100
Technicians	81.6	17.1	0.5	0.9	0	885	100
Protective services	69.8	28.7	0.7	0.4	0.4	1316	100
Para-professionals	51.2	47.6	0.8	0.4	0	1977	100
Office/clerical	81.3	17.4	0.7	0.5	0.2	1896	100
Skilled craft	85.3	13.9	0.3	0.3	0.3	727	100
Service/ maintenance	49.1	49.4	0.8	0.2	0.5	1112	100
Total	72.2	25.5	0.8	1.3	0.2	11167	100
State of D	79.4	16.6	2.3	1.3	0.3	–	100

Source: State of D (1989a)

The Affirmative Action Plan and Program

Apart from an exhortatory policy statement issued in 1989 (State of D 1989b), the state-wide programme exists primarily in the form of the State Governor's Executive Order No. 24 (State of D 1986) which in essence is concerned with providing guidelines rather than the substance of the programme. This is the most recent version of the Affirmative Action Plan first introduced in 1979. Aside from this Executive Order, a substantial state-wide affirmative action programme does not exist; each department and agency within the Executive Branch of government is responsible for drawing up its own plan and to the extent that a state-wide plan exists, it is the summation of these individual efforts. Nonetheless, the effect of Executive Order No. 24 and the organisational responsibilities it establishes is to ensure that affirmative action in pursuit of equal employment opportunity is taken throughout all the departments and agencies of the executive.

The affirmative action and employment equity efforts apply to all 12,000[3] state employees who are subject to the state 'Merit Rules', which in effect constitute the terms and conditions of recruitment, employment, promotion and termination of all non-politically appointed staff (State of D 1987).

Most senior managerial staff – including the State Personnel Director and the Affirmative Action Program Coordinator – are political appointees and hence not covered by the Merit Rules or *ipso facto* affirmative action efforts.

This does not mean, however, that state political appointees do not count in employment equity efforts. Political expediency, if nothing else, will require that the Governor take account of minority interests and sensitivities in the appointments he makes and political expediency may, in this respect, turn out to be a harder taskmaster than formal affirmative action plans.

Affirmative action in practice

There is no statement of the aims of the Affirmative Action Program in Executive Order No. 24 which in all essentials is an affirmation and re-affirmation of commitment to the programme. The Policy Statement issued in December 1989 does contain something more akin to an affirmation of aims but even this is not definitive:

> It is the policy of the State of D to assure equal and fair treatment in all aspects of employment for minorities . . . [and] The principles of an affirmative action program will continue to be specifically followed to ensure that full realisation of equal employment opportunity at all levels of state government employment without regard to race . . . etc.
>
> (State of D 1989b: 1)

Indeed, these aims are unusual in their lack of specificity in respect of what it is hoped to achieve. Any more particular specification of what is to be aimed at is left to the guidance provided for departments in the Executive Order in drawing up their own plans, as we shall see below. The Executive Order lays down the essential components of the individual plans but stipulates that they need not be confined to the items listed. The main components are by now familiar:

- a specific statement of goals and objectives to ensure equal employment opportunities in all aspects of employment;
- specific goals to remedy any under-representation. (There then follows the only allusion to anything approaching a specific goal in the Executive Order. The Order instructs that 'solely' for the purpose of establishing goals and measuring progress towards them, the plan 'shall specify target numbers of minorities . . . and shall include a timetable . . . for meeting the goals. Such numbers shall reasonably reflect the representation of women and minorities in the relevant state-wide labor market' (State of D 1986: II 2.b, A-4).)
- a description of methods proposed for meeting goals including:
    - specific proposals for recruiting minorities,
    - ensuring non-discriminatory hiring practices,
    - equal promotional opportunities,
    - participation in training,
    - career enhancement programmes;
- a proper complaints procedure.

What is of more concern – and interest – however, than these official guidelines is the manner in which they are implemented, because it is at this level that we can begin to understand what the practice of affirmative action involves and what adaptations are made to orthodox merit principles in pursuit of greater minority representation. Though the Executive Order does not specifically stipulate them, each department and agency will prepare workforce, availability and utilisation analyses and, if under-utilisation is shown, will prepare measures for correcting it. Such measures will mostly take the form of outreach activities to schools, colleges, community centres and churches with high proportions of minorities but will also include awareness and sensitivity training for recruiters and interviewers and employment-linked training. These are all orthodox outreach measures and would be easily recognised in Britain. It is in the field of qualifications, testing and selection, however, that departures from orthodoxy are more likely to be found, as we saw in the case of the W police force. So also is it the case in the State of D.

Prior personnel practice (and the Merit Rules) dictated a minimum qualification for each job other than for unskilled jobs. That requirement has been abandoned and no minimum qualification is now stipulated except where it is a genuine occupational qualification as in the case of doctors, engineers and so on. It is now possible, for example, to enter the employ of the state as a social worker on a showing of ability to perform the relevant tasks and without formal qualification. (It remains the case, however, that in order to progress in the profession, it would be necessary to obtain the relevant qualifications. Nonetheless, by abandoning entry qualifications it has been possible to open up the profession to a wider spectrum of aspirants.) During 1989–90 the minimum qualifications required for all 1300 job classifications in the state were revised and measures of a candidate's ability to perform the job based on knowledge, skills and abilities were developed.

In the field of testing, all written tests and examinations are now reviewed at least annually for adverse impact and the use of single tests has been abandoned in favour of a battery of tests for all classes of job. More significantly, in a written response to a report by the Affirmative Action/Equal Employment Opportunity Advisory Council, the State Personnel Office notes that: 'In order to minimise adverse impact, examination passing scores may be adjusted and examination items or components may be revised' (State of D 1990: 1). There is no elaboration on this brief statement and, whilst there is no evidence of systematic race-norming of test scores, it is clear that rigid interpretation of, and adherence to, test scores is relaxed in order to enable more minority candidates to qualify for positions.

All applicants who pass (or satisfy the conditions of) a battery of tests are placed on the 'Certified List' which then constitutes the pool of qualified candidates. In a selection process that closely resembles that used by the W police force, all applicants on the Certified List are put into groups of five with no individual ranking within groups (though the groups themselves will be ranked from 'best' to 'least best'). Placement in a group will be based largely on adjusted scores on the battery of tests but additional 'test points' are given to veterans, thus in effect making veteran status a component of merit (or worthy of compensatory points for disrupted education) and increasing a candidate's chances of being jumped up into a higher group.

Candidates are normally selected from the top group (from within which, there being no individual ranking, choice may be made on a more flexible range of criteria including race)[4] but where under-representation is shown, an agency or department may dip down into the second group. Indeed, one county within the state has legislated to allow minority candidates from a lower group to be brought up into a higher group, thus making them eligible for selection. Majority candidates may not be brought up in this way.

There are a variety of ways, therefore, in which the State of D has adjusted its testing and selection procedures and, in effect, redefined or extended the concept of merit as means of enhancing minority employment and reducing under-representation in the Executive Branch. We shall use a subsequent chapter to discuss whether, and to what extent, these and cognate practices elsewhere have crossed the ill-defined boundary between affirmative action and preferential treatment, and if they have, whether it matters morally speaking. But one final point should be noted. In the absence of time-series data it is not possible to see if and how employment patterns in D are changing. However, what is clear from Table 6.3 is that the pattern of representation of minorities is not just a simple one of under-representation in the higher reaches and over-representation in lower grades. Blacks are over-represented overall while Hispanics (and American Indians) are under-represented. And whilst blacks are over-represented in service and maintenance jobs (as would be expected), this is not the case for Hispanics or Asian-Americans. This complex of patterns will not be changed by the average type of affirmative action plan in the sensitive way required. It is altogether too blunt an instrument for that. The degree of sensitivity of race-conscious programmes is one of the topics that we must return to in later chapters.

THE UNIVERSITY OF DU

For a period stretching over the years 1989–91, the University of DU was engaged in an internal debate about affirmative action practice and its contribution to the creation of a campus with a more diverse faculty, workforce and student body. At the same time that new affirmative action procedures and a revised affirmative action plan were being assembled, there were moves to make these more contributive to the creation of diversity. For many, 'diversity' was of prime importance (as it was – and remains – in many American universities) but even among its strongest proponents there were differing views about whether affirmative action should be an integral part of diversification or a quite separate activity concerned primarily with compliance with federal statutes, orders and regulations. Our discussion of affirmative action at DU University has to be conducted in the context of this internal debate.

In 1989 DU University had a total undergraduate and postgraduate enrolment of 20,477 students, making it the eighth largest of the fifteen major public northeastern universities in the United States (University of DU 1989a: 19, 28). The university receives one quarter of its operating budget from the State of D, the other 75 per cent being made up of grant from the federal government (in virtue of its being a land – and sea – grant institution), from student fees and from private sources. Like other universities it gives preference in admission to students resident in its home state and it exercises a longstanding commitment of service to the communities among which it is located.

The university issued its first affirmative action declaration in 1972 and, although it was more concerned with equal opportunity, equal treatment and non-segregation, this document provided the stimulus for subsequent affirmative action efforts. Another, and more detailed *Equal Employment Opportunity and Affirmative Action Program* was issued in 1986 (University of DU 1986) and this was quickly followed by a substantial revision in 1989 – the *Equal Employment Opportunity and Affirmative Action Program* (Draft) (University of DU 1989b). A month after the new draft programme was issued, a second document appeared under the title *An Overview of the University of DU's Affirmative Action Commitment* (University of DU 1989c). This was presented as a synopsis of the programme '. . . for members of the University community and other persons interested . . .' but substantial parts of its content are not common with the draft programme itself and the two documents appear in parts to be mutually contradictory. A month after the appearance of the *Overview* document an *Ad Hoc* Committee was set up by the University Faculty Senate to review the two draft documents (both of which had been prepared at the direction of the President of the University) and to make recommendations. It was, if anything, the report of this *Ad Hoc* Committee that crystallised the discussion about the relationship of affirmative action procedures to the creation of a more culturally diverse university community. We shall review this debate in more detail later in this section (and the question of diversity will exercise us more in a subsequent chapter) but our current concern is with affirmative action and how it is conducted by the university. It is important to bear in mind, nonetheless, that affirmative action can be seen as primarily an exercise in compliance or as a means to creating greater diversity (see Hacker 1989, Steele 1990a, 1990b, D'Souza 1991).

The aims of affirmative action

Neither the draft *Affirmative Action Program* nor the *Overview* document contain explicit statements of aims, though both make some reference to the value of diversity. It was the view of the university's Affirmative Action Officer, however, that there were three important reasons why affirmative action ought to be pursued. First, it was a means of creating a better representation of minorities – and one that more closely reflected the make-up of the state's population. Second, it would help to create a climate in the university that was more accepting of, and sensitive to, a multi-ethnic and multicultural campus. And third, affirmative action practice itself represents a move away from debate and rhetoric towards practical steps which would in themselves change both attitudes and behaviour on the campus. There was, however, an undeniable (but unstated) sub-theme to these aims which was that the development and implementation of an affirmative action programme were essential for compliance with federal statute and regulation. This must, of course, be a minimum purpose of most affirmative action plans and programmes but what was exercising some people in the university was the extent to which the demands of compliance should dictate the form and reach of affirmative action efforts.

The Affirmative Action Program

The tone of the programme, and its ambiguity of purpose, are set thus:

> The University believes that without the substantial presence of minorities and women in the workforce and student body, the campus community is deprived of the skills and perspectives which are essential to the diversity, balance, and comprehensiveness of a major institution of learning. It is that enriching influence which the University of DU seeks to expand and nurture through its affirmative action efforts.
>
> (University of DU 1989c: 2)

The same document outlines three assumptions which underpin the entire affirmative action process. Two of them are less anodyne than they at first appear. We mention them briefly here because of their prefatory standing to the programme but we shall have reason to return to them in subsequent paragraphs for the broader questions they raise. The first is that no unqualified protected group member must be either hired or promoted. The second is that where there is under-utilisation the first offer of a position must be to a protected class member assuming she or he is qualified. (We shall call this the 'first offer principle'.) The third assumption is that the attributes of the 'best qualified candidate' should include, as well as scholastic (or other relevant) prowess, ability to contribute to diversity and to provide role models for students 'who bring similar qualities to the University'. (This we shall call 'redefining merit'.)

One of the chief barriers to increasing minority representation among faculty and students is – as might be expected from what we have seen in other institutions – the smallness of the availability pool. It is this that tempts institutions to 'recycle' minorities, but it is really a strategy that benefits no-one in the long run. DU, like other universities, has taken the view that if it is to increase minority faculty, then it must nurture its own minority students and groom them for an academic career. This is not made easier, however, by the high drop-out rates among minority students[5] and it is partly in view of this that the university has concentrated much of its affirmative action effort on creating a campus culture that is reassuring for and mindful of the needs of minority students.

Setting goals

Three-year goals are established for each job category within each unit where under-utilisation has been identified. Even where there is no under-utilisation, however, units are encouraged to continue to attract minorities and go beyond 'reasonable representation' in the interests of diversity. (This, at least, is the message given in the university's *Affirmative Action Recruitment Manual* (University of DU undated: 2), though it does not appear in the affirmative action draft programme.)

The goals are set by the deans, directors and administrative department heads and are then submitted to the Affirmative Action Office for approval. In conformity with practice in other institutions, and as we have already noted, the goals relate to all minorities combined – that is, there are not separate goals for different minority groups (even though utilisation data are disaggregated in this way). And, as we would expect, the programme document emphasises that 'The goals are not rigid or inflexible quotas but objectives to be pursued by "good faith effort"'. Neither are they to be used in such a way as to 'grant or deny any individual any employment opportunity because of that individual's race . . .'

Searching and selecting

In conformity with normal equal opportunity practice, all those involved in the hiring process are provided with some training in race and cultural awareness – and most will have been made aware of the university's commitment to diversity. The expectation to increase minority presence among faculty is well established (if not universally approved of).

The principal agent for finding and selecting new faculty is the Search Committee of which, as we have mentioned, the Affirmative Action Officer is an *ex officio* member. The Affirmative Action Officer will endeavour to see that each Search Committee has as diverse a composition as possible, and that they will make every good faith effort to find (and, if possible, hire) minority candidates. This is effected, in theory at least, by requiring every stage of the search and hiring process to be approved by the Affirmative Action Office. In practice, because of resource constraints on the Office, much of this policing has to take the form of scrutiny of paperwork rather than a physical presence on the Search Committee or at interviews.

All documentation concerning the search and hiring process is retained for a period of three years (including a record of the interviews) and is used for periodic internal audits of the personnel process to ensure that all the demands of equal opportunity and affirmative action procedures are complied with in the most effective way. These audits ensure that affirmative action efforts are held under constant review.

First results

It is an axiom of affirmative action that all organisations say that they could do better. To assert anything else is to invite accusations at the very least of complacency, at worst (or almost worst) of complicity in institutional racism. The University of DU is no exception but it also gives strangely conflicting messages. The draft *Affirmative Action Program* identifies a number of specific 'problem areas' concerning minority representation, applicant flows and so on. Thus, two colleges are identified for which minimum applicant flow for minorities is such that without considerable improvement, there would be little hope of increasing minority representation. Second, in the administrative-professional and clerical-technical employment categories, minority employees remain clustered at the lower grades. Third, most academic units under-utilise minority faculty (even, presumably, given the small availability pools) and need to be more aggressive in their affirmative action efforts. And fourth, the hiring rates for minority professionals and support staff had been 'unimpressive'.

The *Overview* document on the other hand paints (albeit very briefly) a more sanguine picture. Commenting on the utilisation data used for setting goals, the *Overview* notes that: 'In general, the University's units are largely in compliance with federal guidelines. The instances of under-utilisation of minority employees and women within specific

EEO-6 job classifications appears to be minimal' (University of DU 1989c: 6). It has to be said that the data on utilisation for each university unit do not support this assertion, but that is not to say that the University of DU is under-utilising minorities to any greater extent than any other university, though there are some that have better established, and more aggressive, affirmative action programmes.[6] The general picture to emerge is one of widespread but not high levels of under-utilisation throughout the university – and with the important exclusion of faculty, there is no reason to believe that energetic affirmative action will not achieve most of the three-year goals.

Qualifications and merit

In common with other institutions we have looked at in America, the most significant aspect of affirmative action at the University of DU in terms of departure from everyday practice – and thus illustrative of the way that affirmative action is changing the rules of the selection and hiring game – is the treatment of the principle of merit and the more flexible interpretation of qualifications. We have already referred to these as they apply to the university's practices as 'redefining merit' and the 'first offer principle'. The latter of these two as it operates in the university is that if the final shortlist of qualified candidates includes a minority group member, then the position should be offered first to this person even if he or she is less qualified than others on the shortlist. It is asserted in the *Overview* document that the university is 'committed' to this practice in order to comply with federal legislation (University of DU 1989c: 7). There is, however, nothing in federal statute, orders or regulations that requires any institution, contractor or otherwise to prefer a less well qualified minority candidate over a better qualified majority candidate. The relevant section of the Uniform Guidelines states that: 'Selection under such [affirmative action] plans should be based upon the ability of the applicant(s) to do the work . . . nor should [the plans] require the selection of persons on the basis of race, color . . . ' etc. (United States Code of Federal Regulations 1989: 41 CFR 60–3.18(4)).

The university plan specifically rules out the hiring of the unqualified and we may therefore assume that the minority candidate selected under the 'first offer principle' will be able to do the work. But insofar as this principle is inconsistent with the practice of hiring 'the best person for the job' who might, as Goldman argues, have 'rights to the position by competence' (Goldman 1979) (which is usually taken to mean the best qualified), then there is a strong prima-facie case (not to say an intuitive assumption) that the 'first offer principle' awards positions at least partly on the basis of 'race and color'.

It is hard to see why the university should wish to claim the protection of federal legislation at all when it could (and does) justify (or at least explain) the use of the 'first offer principle' by redefining what it means to be 'qualified'. The Affirmative Action Officer explained that much depends on what you mean by 'qualified'. In practice, and in his experience, he said it often meant 'being suitable' and 'fitting in' to an organisation, and if qualifications can be thus flexibly interpreted to the benefit of majority candidates then there was no reason why the same should not be the case for minority candidates. (This is a matter we shall take up again in another chapter.) Furthermore, in a community like a university that is trying to promote diversity, a number of other attributes do become relevant in hiring considerations. So, ability to contribute to a diverse community, cultural enrichment, ability to serve minority communities and so on become qualifications. They happen by their nature to be ones that are more likely to be held by candidates who are in the minority. It is an argument, a version of which has been articulated by Dworkin in relation to the *Bakke* and *De Funis* cases (Dworkin 1977a: Chapter 9, 1977b: 11–12), and it is one that is essentially consequence-driven.

Affirmative action and diversity

DU, along with most other universities, has had to engage in some soul-searching about how its affirmative action stance relates to its pursuit of diversity. The discussion has been a relatively recent one even though 'diversity' has been part of university discourse since at least 1978 when the *Bakke* case was decided (*Regents of the University of California v. Bakke* 1978). In his opinion, in that case Justice Powell defended the university's set-aside programme on the grounds that it was being pursued to promote diversity and furthermore that the programme passed the test of 'strict scrutiny' because the pursuit of diversity was the 'compelling' goal that the university was seeking and which (because it *was* 'compelling') satisfied 'strict scrutiny' demands.

The University of DU established its President's Commission to Promote Racial and Cultural Diversity in the Spring of 1988, prior to which it had been little involved in the diversity business. The report of the Commission was published in June 1989 and covered its activities during the period July 1988 to June 1989 and included a list of ten initiatives that should be taken by the university to enhance diversity (University of DU 1989e). These recommendations included that the university should adopt an affirmative action plan (at which stage a final version had not yet been agreed upon). A number of other recommendations concerned the organisation of diversity activities but the remainder identified initiatives that in most respects are barely distinguishable from common affirmative action practices. It appeared that much of what was being recommended in order to pursue diversity differed little from what it was believed ought to be done within an affirmative action programme that was more than just a compliance exercise. And it was this question of the proper and most effective relationship between affirmative action and diversity efforts that generated some soul-searching and not a little heated debate around the turn of the decade. Opinions ranged from those who saw the draft *Affirmative Action Program* as a manifesto for preferential treatment and wanted none of it, to those who wanted a more aggressive programme centred around and incorporating the vigorous pursuit of diversity. In between there were the advocates of separate programmes for affirmative action (as primarily a compliance activity) and for diversity, the purposes of which were quite dissimilar. The Affirmative Action Officer and the Special Assistant to the President were among this last group. And yet, elsewhere, and particularly in the *Ad Hoc* Committee to Review the Affirmative Action Plan, diversity and affirmative action were closely linked, with the latter being a means to the former. So far as this committee was concerned, the university's affirmative action efforts just did not show an adequate dedication to diversity.

Clearly, there *is* a potential conflict of purpose between compliance-directed affirmative action and affirmative action as an integral part of the pursuit of diversity, but if we may trespass briefly into an internal debate of the university, it seems equally clear that the two purposes need not necessarily be in conflict and that the *Ad Hoc* Committee was perhaps puffing pantomime dragon smoke in its strictures against the 'establishment'. The fact is that the university must comply with federal regulations and that affirmative action has to be directed to this end at least as a minimum. There is no reason why it cannot or should not then also serve the ends of diversity. What the *Ad Hoc* Committee was complaining about was that diversity was not put at *the centre* of an affirmative action plan. What it did not consider was whether an affirmative action plan, necessarily tailored to ensure compliance, is the best way of promoting diversity.

There are two other related considerations. The first is what diversity means and what kinds of diversity are involved (elsewhere the *Ad Hoc* Committee refers to low-income groups). Is it to include every conceivable kind of human variation (including abilities, aptitudes and intelligence)? The second is what it means to place diversity as a 'central goal' of 'hiring, pay and promotion policy' (University of DU 1990: 2). The Committee quotes with approval *The Madison Plan* of the University of Wisconsin: 'Our commitment to ethnic diversity is integral to our fundamental commitment to excellence in liberal education' (University of Wisconsin-Madison 1988).

Here, it would seem, the basic functions of a university – academic excellence and scholarship – cannot be fulfilled without diversity. Not only is it central to hiring, pay and promotion in universities, it is at the core of their primary functions. Now it would seem that the criticism that the *Ad Hoc* Committee levelled at the affirmative action plan was, in considerable measure, fuelled by this sort of dedication to the centrality of diversity in the functions of a university. But is not this case for diversity driven more by enthusiasm than wisdom? Might not a more cautionary approach suggest that whilst diversity is to be valued both as an end in itself and as a source of broadening cultural experience on campus, it is *not* central to a university's functions? Was the University of Madison not a centre of excellence in liberal education *before* the diversity movement became the watchword? It does seem that the more enthusiastic case for diversity denies the possibility of fine scholarship before about 1985. That 'ethnic diversity is integral to [a] fundamental commitment to excellence in liberal education' is – to put it no more strongly – a dubious assertion.

THE SA COMPANY

The fourth example of affirmative action practice comes from the private sector. The SA Company is a large chemicals organisation operating on some 250 sites throughout the United States. It is proud of its record of employee relations and of the care it takes of its employees and their families. (Others have called its approach paternalistic.) It has also enthusiastically embraced affirmative action where its efforts have taken it well beyond the strict requirements of federal compliance. It is also keen to promote diversity but for reasons rather different from those of DU University. For SA, diversity is a business necessity. The SA Company, therefore, is an example of a large private sector organisation that has embraced what we have called the 'affirmative action culture' (Edwards 1990b, 1990c). Affirmative action, which has become a part of the personnel process of SA, is pursued only partly (and probably minimally) for compliance purposes and principally as insurance against costly discrimination suits, as means to increasing diversity, and latterly as a response to the changing demographics of the labour force. But perhaps more significantly than any of these, it has become so much a part of everyday practice that its practitioners have almost ceased to articulate any particular reasons for its use.

That affirmative action has taken on a momentum of its own, separate from the demands of compliance, diversity, insurance and demographics, is illustrated by the response of the SA Company when it found that its performance was below that of a number of other chemical corporations. SA meets annually with twenty other chemical companies to compare progress on affirmative action. In 1980, as a result of these meetings, SA discovered that its progress was below the average for all twenty – though in itself, perfectly respectable. This acted as a strong motivator; there was 'pride at stake' and just as if the competition had been over profits, SA wanted to be at the top. The Affirmative Action Committee (at senior management level) therefore decided on an annual target of a 45–50 per cent minority and female intake into management streams for college graduates until SA was at the top of the affirmative action performance list. The target was a crude one; it was not disaggregated into minorities and women. The motivation was simply competitive, and 'fine tuning' took second place to getting results. Within five years SA got the results it wanted; it was at the top of the competition list. It has also created a problem for itself however. After eight years of aggressive affirmative action, it had a relatively large number of minorities and women in lower and middle management who were trapped beneath the 'glass ceiling' and could not progress to senior management. This new situation required that new types of affirmative action for promotion be developed as we shall see.

The affirmative action process

The most difficult recruitment area for SA is with minority scientists. Representation of minorities (and women) in non-professional mana-gerial posts (apart from the glass ceiling problem), and in almost all non-professional, non-managerial posts, has increased markedly over the past decade as a result of aggressive affirmative action and the availability of minorities who could be hired. In the case of scientists (for many of whom a doctorate will be a requirement), no amount of aggressive affirmative action will increase minority representation, simply because the availability pool is so small (at least for black and Hispanic minorities) even given a nationwide search area. In 1990, for example, SA anticipated making nineteen new scientific/engineering appointments requiring a PhD qualification with a minority goal of 20 per cent. In the same year there were sixteen black and Hispanic engineering PhD graduates in the whole of the United States. The company managed to employ one of the four minority PhDs it needed for its goal by headhunting from another company, but despite all its outreach efforts, it did not prove possible to find another three. It had, however, done more than enough to demonstrate good faith efforts. At this level of occupational specialism, therefore, there is little that affirmative action can achieve until the pool of qualified and available minorities is very substantially increased. In the face of this, and to avoid having to compete with other companies for minority staff when they do appear, SA took the decision to create its own pool by funding minority education programmes from schools through to colleges. Some of this is a very long-term investment and depends on generating an early loyalty to SA and maintaining it. The company spent some $1.1 million on such programmes in 1989.

For non-professional staff, outreach takes the usual forms of targeted advertising in the minority press and visits to predominantly minority schools, churches and community centres. These methods have proved to be useful and, on the whole, adequate for positions for which the minority availability pool is not so limited.

Like many other companies of its size, SA goes to very considerable lengths to ensure that all the tests it uses in the hiring and promotion of non-professional staff are as neutral as possible in respect of disparate impact and, where this is not possible, that they are validated for business necessity. The company employs its own expert in testing and she is responsible for ensuring compliance in respect of neutralisation and validation at all sites throughout the United States. This selection specialist shared the view of most other experts in this field that there are no tests that are completely free of disparate impact between different ethnic groups. The SA Company, however, had designed testing procedures which minimised such impact and has invested considerable time and resources in doing so.

There is a further point that must be made here in respect of the use by the company of State Employment Agencies to find new staff and that is that in using such agencies companies like SA may be 'off-loading' their affirmative action responsibilities (and more significantly, responsibility for any preferential treatment) onto the agency. Thus, for example, if a site has ten jobs available and it wishes, for reasons of under-utilisation, to fill three or four of them with minority group members, it may ask the agency to send the appropriate (or more heavily weighted) mix of qualified candidates for interview. Final responsibility for hiring of course remains with the company but it is the agency which must supply not (necessarily) the ten best qualified candidates but the requisite mix of qualified candidates.

We have already noted that the relative success of affirmative action at the managerial levels has created its own problems and necessitated a shift in affirmative action practice itself. Too many minority entrants to management were plateau-ing beneath the 'glass ceiling', having accelerated up the fast track of progression without having been subjected to a sufficiently wide range of training to make further progress possible. Some way had to be found, therefore, to hasten the process of further progression through the glass ceiling. A three-year upward mobility goal was therefore established to push more minority group members into middle management (and some into senior management). To this end, additional training was established along with more mentoring and a reappraisal of attitudes in order to surmount the tendency to greater hesitancy in promoting minorities and women. In respect of them, the question 'Are they really ready yet?' seemed more frequently to be asked than in the case of white males – a situation no doubt exacerbated by their relatively rapid (or assisted) progress through management levels. It remains to be seen whether the 'Glass

Ceiling Commission' established under the 1991 Civil Rights Act will effectively alter this situation.

Qualifications and the merit principle

In previous examples of organisations we have seen that it is in the area of qualifications and what is to constitute qualification that the boundary between affirmative action and preferential treatment becomes most blurred. So it is with SA Company, though there was some reticence in the organisation about the specifics of the treatment of qualifications in the selection procedures. The following sketch provides such details as are available.

First, wherever possible, the idea of what constitutes valuable qualifications is interpreted in fairly broad terms though necessarily including specific subject or professional qualifications for certain positions. Candidates will therefore be assessed on their extra-curricular activities, their leadership abilities and initiative – as measured, for example, by whether they paid their own way through college. Though this broadening of the idea of qualifications to include a variety of personal characteristics is designed to enhance the range of potential candidates (and hence minorities), however, doubts about its efficacy in this regard arise on two fronts. It opens the way to the use of more subjective criteria and judgements which elsewhere in equal opportunities practice are frowned upon as being particularly subject to bias and, unless the wider criteria are carefully selected, they may operate to disadvantage minorities.

Second, when comparing candidates, the idea of the 'best qualified' is no longer used. A number of candidates will normally emerge as 'equally qualified' though on a variable range of qualification criteria. Some may have performed better than others on some criteria and worse on others. As in previous examples we have given, this then allows other, non-strictly job relevant criteria to come into play and, provided there are minority candidates in the 'equally qualified' pool, under-utilisation can be corrected by selecting them. This may be seen as preferential treatment (the only fair way to select between truly equally qualified candidates being by lottery) or as the introduction of utilitarian considerations once the merit principle has exhausted its predictive capacity.

Third, and as a variant on the above, some sites overcome the problem of degrees of qualification and the grading of candidates by the simple expedient of abolishing them and categorising all candidates as either qualified or not qualified. All those in the qualified category are deemed to be equally qualified, and once again, non-merit factors (such as race or gender) may then be used to select successful candidates.

All these processes are designed to enhance the possibilities of selecting minority (and women) candidates for positions. They are all examples of affirmative action; they may also (on some readings at least) constitute preferential treatment. Much revolves around the expedient of abolishing gradations of qualification and counting all qualified (or, in previous cases, all within a group of five or so) candidates as equally qualified. Technically speaking this rules out the possibility of a white male candidate claiming that he has been passed over for a less well qualified minority candidate. It is also argued that systematically (or at least regularly) choosing the black or Hispanic candidate in these circumstances is in principle no different from the decades of systematic bias to white males. The moral dubiety of this last argument is self-evident *unless* it is being proposed as an argument for compensation. It does seem that the process of re-designing the merit principle is in pursuit of assisting (or preferring) minorities and that the rationale implicit in the final selection represents a substitution of utility for fairness (unless again, preference is defended on grounds of compensation). We shall discuss these matters further in a subsequent chapter.

Affirmative action results

It was not possible to obtain detailed time-series information on minority representation in SA. The following figures give recent general trends. The ethnic and sex composition of the workforce varies enormously between its constituent businesses and sites. Progress at professional and supervisory levels has been most marked in the 'chemicals and specialities' businesses where the percentage of the workforce who were from minority ethnic groups increased from 5.9 per cent in 1980 to 8.7 per cent in 1987. The oil division registered a small decrease in minority representation between 1985 and 1987 from 9.1 per cent to 8.9 per cent, and over the same period the coal division registered a slight increase but from a very low baseline of 1.7 per cent to 1.9 per cent. In the company as a whole, however, by 1989 minorities represented 6.3 per cent of *middle* and *upper* management, a figure that was seen to represent the success of affirmative action activities (SA Company 1989: 3).

Diversity

The SA Company is no exception to the obeisance paid to diversity, though in its case it is more a matter of perceived self-interest than the fetishisation that is apparent in some universities. Even so, its assertions that diversity is good for business seem to owe more to the current popularity of the concept than to hard analyses of the benefits that might flow from it. Perhaps it is rather a matter that large companies cannot afford for the sake of their public image *not* to be seen to be embracing diversity.

There were a number of components to the 'good for business' argument put by several people within SA. First, diversity was seen to be a value worth nurturing because of the variety of skills, talents and viewpoints it brought into the company. This diversity of talent and culture was 'the only advantage we have over some of our competitors such as the Japanese'. Second, it was argued that SA did not always want to remain primarily an American company; it has global aspirations. A diverse workforce and a diverse outlook therefore were essential in this enterprise – not least because SA's customers would be increasingly diverse and the company must be sensitive to their requirements. Third, diversification of the workforce was a necessary response to demographic changes. In common with most other large enterprises, SA has seen the need to turn to diversity if it is to maintain a qualified workforce (or indeed a workforce), given that over the decade 1990–2000 80–85 per cent of net additions to the workforce will be minorities and women and that by 2025 minorities will comprise 40 per cent of college-age youth (see Hudson Institute 1987, 1988).

An ethnically diverse workforce will therefore be an inevitability and a diversity programme is simply making a virtue out of necessity. It is not unreasonable to think therefore that SA (in common with most companies) would not have embraced diversity had it not been faced with the inevitability of demographic change. Nor is it unreasonable to argue that the current rhetoric about cultural diversity owes at least something to the need to lend an air of moral rectitude to what is in reality a necessary response to the inevitable.

Where then does affirmative action fit into this drive for diversity and has SA faced the same dilemmas that we identified at the University of DU? The answer to the latter is 'seemingly not', and in respect of the former, the company has for many years pursued affirmative action well beyond the limits of what is required for compliance. The same programmes and procedures that were (and are) used for compliance (and beyond compliance) now serve in the pursuit of diversity. There is no organisational divergence between the two activities and the affirmative action that was aggressively pursued for public relations and competitive motives is just the same activity that pursues diversity.

It has been the purpose of these brief sketches to provide some of the 'feel' of affirmative action practice in a variety of institutions in America and Great Britain. What happens in practice clearly often diverges from 'official' accounts and both will have to inform our subsequent discussion.

7 Practice compared
Britain and America

Reduced to its basic element, the purpose of affirmative action is universally common – to shift the balance of burdens and benefits between morally arbitrarily defined groups in society. Again, reduced to essentials, affirmative action is simply one policy tactic to bring this about. These basics are common to both the countries surveyed in foregoing chapters but beyond the basics there is considerable variation engendered by the different demographic and social contexts within which affirmative action operates. We use this chapter to point up some of the similarities – but mainly the differences – in affirmative action purpose and practice between Great Britain and the United States. Some, though not all, of these will have a bearing on the potential effectiveness of the practice.

THE EFFECTS OF AFFIRMATIVE ACTION

Of the fifteen organisations in Great Britain and the United States practising some form of affirmative action that we examined in earlier chapters, eight attributed minority increases among employees in general, and upper grades in particular, to their affirmative action activities or components of these activities. None were able to prove a connection between affirmative action and increased minority representation however. For two of these eight, adequate time-series data to show minority increases were not available but respondents were confident nonetheless that their affirmative action (and in the case of the W police, its preferential treatment) were having a beneficial effect. In the case of DU University, the Affirmative Action Office was not in possession of sufficient time-series data to demonstrate incontrovertibly the effect of its three-year plan, but was confident nonetheless that on (then) current evidence the plan's goals would be reached within three years except in the case of faculty members. The SA Company was having mixed results but considered that its affirmative action efforts had been responsible for getting minorities into 6.3 per cent of middle and upper management posts.

The results in C local authority in Great Britain suggest what might be more broadly true (though evidence is insufficient to test it soundly), that the drawing up and implementation – with deadlines – of an affirmative action plan may be of less importance in itself than more general attitudes and policies about minorities in an organisation. In C there had been big increases in minority representation between 1984 and 1989 (an increase of 51.9 per cent) – that is, before a new and aggressive affirmative action plan was introduced in 1989/90. Having a 'plan' does help to focus activity and gain results but it is not a necessary vehicle for success.

Two organisations, the KX Company and A local authority, both in Great Britain, whilst having relevant data, could not produce evidence that their affirmative action efforts were producing the desired results. For five other organisations, the time-series data that are necessary to monitor the composition of the workforce were not kept or were not available or were too inadequate. For these organisations, it is not possible to say whether their affirmative action efforts are yielding success or not.

The statistical data are inadequate to the task of accurately measuring changes in the representation of different minority groups among institutions' employees. Even less has it proved possible, where change data are available, to attribute changes in minority representation unequivocally to affirmative action efforts. (We must allow for the possible effects of a number of other variables which may range from unrelated changes in personnel practice to demographic change in the labour draw area.)

What is of more value, however, from our examination of these fifteen organisations, is the evidence about the variety of affirmative action practices that they pursue. This is of particular interest when we compare practices in the two countries (we have already noted that there is a fairly standard package of practices – but with variations – in Britain). There is (as would be expected) a good deal of overlap between British and American practice but the latter shows some very marked differences. It is not just the degree of sophistication (as in neutralising tests and so on) that marks out American practice; more importantly, there is the clear evidence of what we have already maintained – that race-conscious practice in the United States has shifted quite markedly towards the preferential treatment end of the continuum.

DEMOGRAPHIC AND SOCIAL CONTEXTS

There is one simple fact that is usually overlooked when comparisons are made between affirmative action in Britain and America and which is, I believe, of signal importance to the manner in which it is pursued.

Ethnic minorities make up 5.5 per cent of the population of Great Britain but 26 per cent of the population of the United States. It matters less that there are geographical concentrations in each country which push local 'minority' representation much higher than these global figures, than that the global figures themselves must in part set the tone and level of governmental concern and policy. Quite simply, it makes a big difference to the extent to which race matters rise up the government's agenda of concern whether it is a quarter of the population that is affected, or only a little over a twentieth. The sheer nastiness and hurt of racial bigotry is not altered by the numbers affected, but it would be naive to think that government concern is unrelated to the magnitude of the problem. It should not surprise us, therefore, that affirmative action is not pursued with as much vigour in Great Britain as in America, or that legislation in the latter country makes much greater demands on both public and private sector employers than it does in the former. (And since, in the febrile state of race relations debate in Britain, this will be interpreted as condoning racism, I hasten to add that it is simply a statement of fact.)

There are other matters, related to the proportionate size of the minority groups, which will affect the climate within which race-conscious issues are debated of course – such as the numbers and types of minorities, the length of time for which they have constituted a part of the population, and the history of prejudice, discrimination and bigotry that they have suffered. A detailed discussion of these goes beyond the scope of this book, however, and insofar as the promotion of affirmative action practices is concerned, it may well be that the proportionate size of the minorities in the population is, if not the most, then among the most important demographic factors.

Affirmative action, though often seen as one component of employment policy (though with business contract set-asides it has other features as well), does not operate in a social policy vacuum. Thus, while the very different welfare arrangements that exist in Great Britain and the United States (see, for example, Higgins 1978) might have little direct impact on the form that affirmative action takes in these countries, the nature and extent of welfare provision will, of course, affect the relative social and economic conditions of minorities, and hence the consequences for them if affirmative action does not work or does not work well. To this extent then, the costs of failure may be less severe in Great Britain than in the United States. This is not to suggest that affirmative action is in any substantive sense an alternative to welfare provision, but there is some evidence (though as yet patchy) that affirmative action in the United States has contributed to an increasing inequality *within* some minority groups (and particularly African-Americans) by providing a ladder for some whilst leaving others to inadequate and stigmatising welfare (see Sowell 1990, Steele 1990b, Bolick 1990, Claiborne *et al.* 1983).

MOTIVES

Employers in the United States undertake affirmative action because they have to. In Great Britain they do it voluntarily (those that do do it). However, many employers in America do far more than they need to for compliance purposes and in all likelihood would continue with it even if compulsion were removed. Compulsion in itself, therefore, is a contributory but not an adequate explanation of the prosecution of affirmative action.

Apart from compulsion, there is a wide mix of motives for conducting affirmative action, some explicit, some unstated, some rhetorical, some self-delusional. But the mix of motives does vary as between our two countries (and, it would seem, the degree of self-delusion or cynicism). Thus, in Great Britain, where compulsion cannot be claimed as the bottom-line reason for affirmative action, we have to look elsewhere for the 'real' motive for its use. In the public sector this may well lie in political or ideological reasons and be couched in the rhetoric of anti-racism, equal opportunity and equality (but not necessarily any the less 'genuine' for being rhetorical). Or it may – as seems also the case in the United States – be a service-provision argument that the providers of services ought to reflect in their ethnic (and gender) make-up, the composition of the communities they serve. (This, it should be noted, is, morally speaking, quite a different argument to the more apodictic one that for reasons of justice and equity – not service – the composition of local government workforces ought to reflect that of their labour draw area.)

In the private sector in Great Britain, the 'good for business' argument appears to have taken hold notwithstanding that there is as yet little evidence to support the contention that an ethnically mixed (or 'representative') workforce is more productive, innovative, efficient or profit-producing. No doubt this has much to do with the need to 'sell' equality of opportunity and affirmative action within the company – and particularly to senior management. Whatever image a company wishes to present (and being an 'equal opportunity employer' may increasingly be a part of a corporate image), an appeal to self-interest could well be a more productive approach for a personnel manager to take internally than one that tries to stake out the moral high ground of justice and equity.

Similar arguments no doubt apply in America but, as we have seen, the debate about affirmative action there, in both public and private sectors, appears to have been overlaid in recent years by the new enthusiasm for diversity.[1] To the extent that this has happened, it reflects a shift in the moral grounds of argument. Affirmative action has in the past been defended (in both public and private sectors, but more so in the former than the latter) on grounds of justice. Either it has been unjust not to provide equality of opportunity, or past harm has required present compensation. Diversity, on the other hand – at least on the evidence presented here – is much more likely to be promoted on grounds of utility – or at least consequence. Thus a diverse student and faculty body is necessary for sound liberal scholarship; diversity is good for business (again); a diverse workforce will be more sensitive to an increasingly diverse market; diversity brings innovative ideas and so on. What remains puzzling, however, is how much of this is true and how much of it is genuinely believed. And if the answer is 'not much' in both cases, why is affirmative action seemingly pursued with a vigour that often goes beyond the demands of compliance?

The remaining argument is the demographic one. Affirmative action in pursuit of a more diverse workforce is simply a response to the inevitable. There is some logic in this but it does not provide the whole answer. If an increasing proportion of the labour force will be drawn from minority groups and if the level of qualifications and expertise among these groups is not adequate to satisfy your employment needs, then it makes sense to train and mentor and nurture (all forms of 'outreach'). But beyond that, where high levels of qualification are not required, there seems little point in working aggressively to employ more minorities (other, that is, than for moral reasons) if perforce they will appear anyway because of their greater representation in the population and labour force.

PROPORTIONALITY, REPRESENTATION AND AVAILABILITY

Whether or not goals are set, most establishments have some conception, however vague, of what the minority ethnic composition of their workforce 'ought' to be. Among contractor establishments in the United States goals must be set where there is under-utilisation of minorities. In Great Britain, the setting of goals, as part of the affirmative action process, will be a voluntary matter and a number of the establishments in Britain that we looked at in an earlier chapter did not set goals. There is an important difference, however, both conceptually and technically in the nature of the goals set as between Great Britain and America. In Great Britain, where there is no official guidance on these matters, the nature of the goals set (by those establishments that do set them) is in consequence more diverse. Among the establishments described earlier, some set goals that used some approximation to representation in the labour draw area, some that used minority representation in the city or county, some that were aiming for a reflection of minority representation in the population of Britain as a whole, and two in which goals bore some resemblance to those required in the United States. These last two examples apart, however, what is common to all the goal setting we have described in Great Britain is that it is directed towards an end result in which the minority representation in the workforce is the same (or approximately the same) as that in some defined population as a whole (draw area, city, county or nation). On the assumption, therefore, that this is not just a purely quixotic or arbitrary end-state to be achieved (or – and there is probably more substance in this assumption – that it is simply the easiest target to aim for) we must surmise that this state of affairs is considered to be the 'right' one insofar as it would constitute the nature of things in a world devoid of discrimination, racial prejudice and racial deprivation. In short, in the absence of these things, all minorities would be distributed both horizontally and vertically across the reward system of jobs, statuses and positions in proportion to their presence in the defined population. When articulated in such a way, however, such an assertion draws instant denials and claims that no one holds to so simplistic an assumption. And that is probably true, but the fact is that 'similar proportions' remains the only underlying logic of the sorts of goals that *are* predominant in Great Britain.

We have to contrast this state of affairs with the availability analyses required of federal contractors in the United States. Earlier chapters have described how the goals that are set within affirmative action programmes in the United States are determined by levels of under-utilisation which in turn are a measure of the disparity between current minority representation in the workforce and their estimated 'availability' in the relevant labour force. Availability, however, as calculated by the eight-factor analysis, bears little relation to what in Britain would be called 'representation'. The latter is (usually) a simple measure of the proportion of the population – or sometimes the proportion of the working age population – in a given area that comes from minority ethnic groups. Availability on the other hand is a measure of the numbers (or sometimes the proportions) of minority group members who are available for work and qualified or trainable for a particular type of job. Given an adequate availability pool, therefore, and vacancies to fill, there is little reason for continued under-utilisation, assuming that minority people wish to take up that type of employment. This is not the case with representation, which provides no indication of the numbers or proportions of minority group members who *would* be in a position to take up and carry out any particular type of job were it available.

The technical differences between goals based on representation and those based on availability are evident. The conceptual implications are less immediately obvious. Availability provides a more accurate (and reasonable) estimate of the numbers and proportions of minorities that an employer ought to have in his workforce in the absence of all discriminatory barriers and assuming no significantly different pattern of career and job choices as between minority groups, and between them and the majority. But the assumption behind availability measures is that these are the numbers and proportions of minorities an employer ought to have, *given* the historic pattern of discrimination, prejudice and bigotry. In other words, availability allows the costs of past harm to lie where they fall; it accepts as a given the present consequences of past discrimination. To this extent, therefore, goals based on availability measures contain no element of compensation for past harm; they do not state what the representation of minorities in any given job type or occupation ought now to be had past discrimination *not* occurred.

Now whilst goals based on crude minority representation in the population contain some pretty heroic assumptions about why these should be replicated in workforces, and whilst in almost all instances in which they are used it is for reasons of convenience (and the lack of ready availability of alternatives), they do at least, if only by default, include some element of counterfactual reasoning. And this is because, whatever the proportion of minorities in workforces would now be had past discrimination not occurred, it is a reasonable assumption that it would be nearer to representation in the labour force (if not the population as a whole) than it would to current availability with its in-built 'acceptance' of the consequences of past discrimination.

QUALIFICATIONS AND MERIT

It is a matter of fine judgement whether a more flexible approach to the use of qualifications or a reformulation of what constitutes merit count as affirmative action or preferential treatment. It seems almost certainly to be the case that the examples described in foregoing chapters would not have been introduced had it not been for the need or desire to increase minority representations. What is less clear is whether members of the majority population are disadvantaged by such practices. It may on the one hand be argued that if the relaxed (or different) use of qualifications and merit apply equally to all candidates, then no preference is being given to minorities. But against this it may be said that if on more traditional interpretations of qualification or merit white candidates would have been appointed to positions that now go to minority candidates on a different interpretation, then much hinges on the nature of these alternative interpretations. And if the 'relaxed' interpretation has been designed specifically to enable more minorities to be appointed, then there is a prima-facie case for saying that majority candidates have been disadvantaged. But these are arguments that we shall take up at greater length in another chapter.

Practice in the United States is a long way further down the road in terms of the reinterpretation of qualifications and merit as an affirmative action tactic than is the case in Great Britain and this no doubt is a reflection of the length of time that affirmative action has been practised there and the vigour with which it has been pursued. One of the private sector organisations in Britain that have been described here had adopted a practice of substituting relevant experience for professional or academic qualifications where this was feasible, and no doubt marginal adjustments to the use of qualifications are being made in many other private and public sector organisations, but there is no evidence that the systematic (and quite fundamental) changes that have come about in American practice are anywhere evident in British practice.

THE POOL

The determining limitation to the effectiveness of affirmative action, even when aggressively pursued, is the size of the availability pool. If qualified and available minorities do not exist in sufficient numbers then no amount of affirmative action other than that which concentrates on training will increase their representation in workforces. It is in large measure because of the limited pool that affirmative action practice in the United States has become ever more inventive in the ways that we have described earlier. It seems unlikely, however, that inventiveness can be pushed much further without becoming overtly and extensively preferential. The situation in Great Britain is rather more complicated for two reasons. First, no-one knows what the availability pool is for any given job type, because no one has measured availability with the degree of sophistication used in America. A measure of representation in the population will, for reasons already explained, produce a much higher target figure than will availability and thus give the impression of much higher levels of under-representation. But overall minority representation in the population (or even in the labour market) cannot be treated as a measure of the pool of available minorities and to the extent that it is, then we are dealing with a different conception of what constitutes a 'pool'.

The second complication in Great Britain is that the two main groups of minorities, the Afro-Caribbean and the Asian (but with significant sub-group differences within the latter – see Brown 1984), have very divergent educational experiences and career expectations. The 'pool problem' will be very different therefore as between these two groups.[2]

It is difficult therefore to assess the extent to which minority under-representation in Britain is to be explained by the lack of qualified (or potentially qualified) minorities as against other factors such as discrimination and occupational choices. Certainly, none of the British establishments discussed in an earlier chapter volunteered a limited pool as a significant limiting factor in their attempts to increase minority representation in their workforces, but at the same time most were finding it necessary to use a variety of training schemes to enhance the number of qualified minorities; and evidence from elsewhere suggests that non-availability is a barrier to increased representation. The Metropolitan Police Force, for example, has for more than a decade identified inadequate qualifications among minority candidates as one (but by no means the only) reason for their under-representation (see Timmins 1982, Helm 1987, *Personnel Management* 1990, Oakley 1988). Notwithstanding this evidence, however, we have a much clearer picture of the nature and extent of the pool problem in America, if for no other reason than the greater informativeness of proper availability data and utilisation analyses. And if it *is* the case that a limited availability pool is a more significant barrier to further progress in the United States, this may have much to do with the fact that affirmative action has been pressed harder and further there than in Great Britain. It could well be the case, therefore, that if affirmative action were pursued more aggressively (and extensively) in Britain and were to be accompanied by more sophisticated availability analyses, it would become necessary to reassess the relative impacts of pool size and discrimination as limiting agents to further progress, with a higher weighting having to be given to the former.

SENIORITY

As with most of the problems attendant on the use of affirmative action and for reasons primarily to do with the length of time for which it has been pursued, seniority exercises more concern in the United States than in Great Britain. Protecting affirmative action gains from the disproportionate effects of using length of service as a criterion for redundancy may be a problem for some equal opportunities units in Great Britain, but it has certainly not attained the practical or symbolic importance that it has in America. The seniority question has been tested by two notable cases in the Supreme Court (*Firefighters Local 1785 v. Stotts* 1984, *Wygant v. Jackson* 1986) and it has been the subject of extensive discussion elsewhere (see, for example, Fiscus 1992, Kirp and Weston 1987, Levin-Epstein 1987).

The moral issues raised by these debates will be examined in a later chapter; our purpose here is simply to note that whilst seniority and the protection of affirmative action gains may exercise a number of employers in Great Britain, it is not a matter that has tested the morality of affirmative action as has been the case in America.

THE STANDING OF AFFIRMATIVE ACTION

There a number of dimensions on which affirmative action may have significance. Amongst the more obvious are politics, equal opportunity practice, personnel practice more generally, race relations and the debate about race relations in the social policy arena, and not least in the field of moral or social philosophy. It will not be our purpose to survey all of these but rather, more briefly, to highlight the main differences in the standing of affirmative action between America and Great Britain.

Affirmative action finds its way onto the political agenda (but always somewhere near to 'any other business') in Britain only very infrequently and then only in the context of an incident of civil unrest or, more likely, of some pursuant report that will catalogue racial deprivation and discrimination, point to institutionalised racism in the education system, bemoan the rich ethnic cultures that the country is failing to profit by and then prescribe affirmative action as an urgent necessity but only for a limited time and never, never, 'positive discrimination' or quotas. Subsequent debate will concentrate on the evils of positive discrimination and quotas.[3] In short, the intellectual sophistication of the debate in Britain has not advanced since the 1970s when 'positive discrimination' first entered the political lexicon (see Edwards 1987: Chapters 1, 2). 'Positive action' and 'positive discrimination' remain part of the padding in the rhetoric of race-talk. For these reasons, the moral questions attached to affirmative action (and preferential treatment), and their place in social policy practice more generally, have never received a proper airing. What has changed, however, since the late 1970s is the greater 'normalisation' of affirmative action within equal opportunities and personnel practice. This is still a long way short of its incorporation into practice (and culture) in the United States but 'affirmative action' does now refer to a fairly standard and agreed set of practices among practitioners in Great Britain. It remains, nonetheless, a voluntary practice, pursued for a variety of reasons (some of which possibly owe more to self-deception or the strictures of a liberal orthodoxy than to moral prescription or proven self-interest) and always vulnerable, because of the absence of compulsion, to the vicissitudes of political and economic change. But once again we have to ask whether we would (or should) expect a policy practice that is designed to serve the interests of perhaps no more than 5 per cent of the population to take a more central and substantive part in political debate and in social policy practice.

In Northern Ireland – the only part of the UK where affirmative action is mandatory – it is, because of its youth, a very fragile animal and it is not unreasonable to think that if compulsion were removed, it might disappear as quickly as it arrived. Such is not the case in America.

Some (perhaps many) smaller contractors would drop affirmative action plans were Executive Order 11246 to be rescinded, but there is sufficient evidence to indicate a strong possibility that most public agencies, most universities and colleges, and most large companies would continue with affirmative action even if all compulsion were removed. There are many reasons for this, but three are, I think, paramount. The first is demographic necessity, though how 'real' a reason this is it is hard to say. As we pointed out earlier, if minorities are going to constitute an increasing part of the labour force, there seems little need to develop affirmative action outreach measures to find them. Second, 'diversity' is increasingly taking over as the main *asserted* reason for pursuing affirmative action. But as we have seen, there is a high 'froth factor' in diversity-talk so that isolating motives for action is particularly difficult. Nor is this made easier by the fact that 'diversity' has taken on some of the complexion of a moral crusade. Whatever the motives behind it however (self-interest, commercial considerations, conformity to politically correct orthodoxy, a desire for justice) it seems, for the moment at least, to be unstoppable. But even if diversity had not entered the scene, it seems likely (albeit at a conjectural level) that affirmative action would survive the removal of compulsion. This can be attributed to our third reason – that affirmative action has become a part of the 'culture' of equal opportunities and personnel practice, particularly in larger companies and in the public sector as we showed in Chapter 6 and as I have argued elsewhere (Edwards 1990c). Many of the practices that we have identified as constituting affirmative action, including race-proofing all selection procedures, neutralising tests, reassessing qualifications and merit and a variety of outreach efforts, are now standard practice; they are what is normally done. For most establishments, the financial investment has been made in them and to abandon them now would require a purposeful reversal of policy, writing off that investment rather than simply dropping inconvenient ways with no cost implications. Furthermore, to abandon affirmative action now would not be to revert to 'normal' practice; it has been in place long enough to *be* normal practice. To do away with affirmative action now would be tantamount to a decision to revert to old fashioned, out-of-date and outmoded personnel practices. In short, affirmative action has gained an inertial momentum in the United States which for many (probably most large) companies makes compulsion irrelevant (see Dwyer 1989). It is this, more than anything else, that distinguishes the practice in America from that in Great Britain.

PREFERENTIAL TREATMENT

On a number of occasions in describing affirmative action practices, we have noted how a particular practice might cross the inexact boundary between affirmative action and preferential treatment. The locus of this boundary and the relative moral standing of the two types of practice will be the subject of extended treatment in a later chapter, but we shall complete the present chapter with what need be only a brief word about preferential treatment and affirmative action in Britain and America.

The moral rectitude of affirmative action and the iniquity of preferential treatment have been the stuff of official comment and academic and political debate in both countries. Nowhere is preferential treatment officially sanctioned (other than as court-ordered remedy in America). In Great Britain such debate as there is about affirmative action remains stubbornly bogged down in assertions of preference as we have already noted. And in the United States there is a strong body of opinion (amongst which African-Americans are strongly represented) that remains staunchly opposed to practices of preference. But what is *done* in these two countries differs very markedly. It would be naive to assume that preferential treatment does not happen in Great Britain, though its extent is impossible to judge. Certainly, some of the evidence described earlier suggests that some affirmative action practices may be such as to produce a bias in favour of minorities and that others are informally implemented to create the same effect. Much, of course, will depend on whether one sees affirmative action as correcting a previously unjust balance or as a departure from purely ethnically neutral merit criteria. What can be said with certainty is that the magnitude of preferential treatment in Great Britain is infinitesimal compared with the United States. In America it is common and widespread. The examples given earlier showed that the shift from affirmative action to preferential treatment can be easy and imperceptible. It happens in two ways: rules, regulations and criteria can be amended or rewritten in such a way as to allow more minorities to qualify for consideration (which may not in itself, as we have already noted, be preferential); and selection processes may be tailored in such a way as to enable a minority person to be chosen (as when several candidates are all defined as equally qualified and a minority candidate chosen from among them on non-merit criteria), which almost certainly conforms with what most would conceive of as preferential treatment. (It is worth noting in this respect that in *Texas Department of Community Affairs v. Burdine*, the Supreme Court, whilst acknowledging that an employer has discretion to choose between equally qualified candidates provided the choice is not based on unlawful criteria, noted that Title VII neither demands preferential treatment nor *requires* that employment practices be altered in order to maximise minority or female employment. This may reasonably be read as indicating that whilst Title VII does not require changes in employment practice, neither does it proscribe them.[4] The sorts of changes to selection procedures that we have noted earlier therefore may be permitted by Title VII, but much will then hinge on whether the final selection criteria are lawful or not (*Texas Department of Community Affairs v. Burdine* 1981).

Why, then, if preferential treatment is unlawful is it allowed to happen – and on what appears to be a large scale? (We make no judgement here about whether it *should* be unlawful or not.) The answer I believe lies in the fact that the proscription of preferential treatment both in Title VII of the Civil Rights Act 1964 and in the Code of Federal Regulations is a proscription of *quotas in terms*. To forbid preferential treatment as such would be a much more difficult task definitionally. To distinguish quotas from goals is a relatively easy task; clearly to separate affirmative action from preferential treatment is well nigh impossible, particularly in legal terms. Provided, therefore, that employers steer clear of quotas, which most do, there remains very considerable latitude within which to extend activity into preferential treatment with impunity. But there is much more to be said on this matter.

8 The moral dilemmas of preference

On 23 January 1989 the Supreme Court decided *City of Richmond v. J.A. Croson Company* on appeal from the Fourth Circuit Court of Appeals. Five and a half months later, on 4 June it decided *Ward's Cove Packing Company v. Frank Atonio.* These two cases, one an affirmative action case, the other concerning a complaint of discrimination, lay at the centre of what was interpreted by most proponents of affirmative action as a concerted attack by a conservative Supreme Court on the practice, and led, two years later, as we have seen, to the enactment of a new Civil Rights Act. But neither the Court's decisions in these (and other) cases, nor the new Act, resolved what are now some longstanding moral questions about affirmative action and preferential treatment. The doubts entertained by a majority of the Court (Justices Rehnquist, O'Connor, White, Scalia and Kennedy in both cases) reflected some of these moral concerns and, in particular, a desire to see the benefits of affirmative action confined to actual victims, a desire to pull back from correcting for 'general social discrimination', and a determination to halt practices that might (not just would) involve the setting of quotas. The quiet consensus about the move from affirmative action to preference practices that had developed throughout the 1980s had, it seemed, been challenged. The Court's decisions and accompanying opinions, however, were informed more by a determination to rein in affirmative action than by a desire to weigh means against moral ends. (It was left to the four dissenting justices to draw attention to why affirmative action was being taken in the first place.) The decisions, in short, generated more heat than illumination and the moral dilemmas of preference remain unresolved.

The matters discussed in this chapter are the principal unresolved questions concerning the moral standing of preference policies which we take to be the 'hard' end of a continuum of which soft affirmative action is the other. As long ago as 1975, Nathan Glazer was complaining that the affirmative action of the Executive Orders had, in its interpretation under the 1964 Civil Rights Act, become the imposition of 'proportionate representation'. He notes that: '[Affirmative action] assumes that everyone is guilty of discrimination; it then imposes on every employer the remedies which in the [Act] could only be imposed on those guilty of discrimination' (Glazer 1975: 58). The claim that affirmative action had moved into the realm of preferential treatment and the original aim of equality of opportunity had become one of creating 'statistical parity' became a common theme amongst those who saw the original purposes and methods of affirmative action thwarted by the urgent drive to achieve proportionality. Thus, Abram has argued that the proponents of equal opportunity (the 'fair shakers') have been ousted by the 'social engineers' who impose quotas and use preference whilst calling them goals and affirmative action (Abram 1986); Capaldi traces the cycle of race-conscious policies from 'Jim Crow' laws to 'reverse discrimination' and sees in this the hand of 'doctrinaire liberalism' (Capaldi 1985); Lynch, in somewhat overheated prose, refers to the shift from equality of opportunity to a 'racial spoils system' and the emergence of a 'new McCarthyism' which brands all who dare to speak out against affirmative action as racists (Lynch 1989); and Sowell and Steele (both blacks) have in more temperate language bemoaned the harm that is being done to African-Americans by the implications of inferiority that lie beneath the assumed need for preferential treatment (Sowell 1975, 1977, Steele 1990a, 1990b).

But one has to be neither proponent nor opponent of policies of preference to acknowledge the fact that there *has* been a shift in policy over the past two decades. There *is* an element of disingenuousness among those who continue to call current practices 'affirmative action' as if they differed not at all from what was originally meant by the term. Much better to call them what they often are – preferential treatment – and then confront the moral dilemmas head on rather than pretend they are something they are not. After all, there are moral grounds for a defence of preferential treatment and they need to be aired before we can judge whether they are sufficiently compelling. That practice itself has changed, there can be little doubt; the examples provided in Chapter 6 are illustrative of more widespread practice as attested to in the diversity programmes of many universities and the acknowledged employment policies of many large companies and of federal, state and local agencies. Aggressive affirmative action that slides almost imperceptibly into preferential treatment is characteristic of the 'affirmative action culture' that we have described earlier.

There is no escaping the fact, therefore, that the moral debate about affirmative action must also necessarily be a debate about the moral standing of policies of preference. Earlier evidence has shown that whilst theory may delineate a clear boundary between affirmative action and preferential treatment, practice acknowledges no such distinction. And whilst the law proscribes *quotas in terms* it does not do the same for preferential treatment – indeed cannot do so until someone defines it.

Letting merit alone count, therefore, can now mean letting race count; abandoning rigid and small differences in qualifications can open the way to using non-merit criteria; 'creating diversity' can compete with 'best qualified for the job'; and goals when subjected to the imperatives of the 'affirmative action culture' can become quotas. Preference, then, is widespread in America; what is less clear (though not entirely unclear) is why it has become so, but there would appear to be two dominant reasons. The first we have already aired – the in-built momentum of the affirmative action culture. The second is related. It is that affirmative action has probably raised expectations beyond a level to which the practice itself can deliver. As we have seen, the greatest limitation on increasing minority representation, particularly in occupations requiring higher qualification levels, is the inadequacy of the availability pool. There are only a limited number of ways around this *impasse*; one, as we have seen, is 'poaching' or 'recycling' qualified minorities, but this can only be of very limited value for obvious reasons. Two, potentially more productive ways are to wait for the education system to produce more qualified minority group members – a slow and uncertain process – or to circumvent the limited pool by using preference practices. Having started down this latter road by investing heavily in affirmative action, there must be a great temptation to take the additional steps into preference to achieve the results that past investment has so far denied. After all, good faith efforts may satisfy the OFCCP but only tangible results will repay the investment that many agents, both public and private, have made in affirmative action. And the goal-directed behaviour of the affirmative action culture is instrumental rather than affective; satisfaction comes with results not with having done your best.

EXTRA EFFORT VERSUS PREFERENCE PRACTICE

In the areas of employment (including hiring and promotion), while goals may be distinguished from quotas in a legalistic sense, the ideal-type distinction between affirmative action and preferential treatment would appear to be that while the former, whilst making extra efforts, ceases to operate at the point of hiring or promotion and allows merit and merit alone to decide who should succeed, the latter may continue to operate at the point of decision and, in doing so, override merit (and violate the merit principle). Once more, and for the purposes of the present arguments only, we shall treat the merit principle as uncontestable (which it is not, as subsequent discussion shows) and simply assert that the idea of hiring and promoting by merit and only merit is deemed to bestow upon the most meritorious a *right* to the position for which he or she is in competition. When we say, therefore, that preferential treatment overrides the merit principle, we are saying that it violates people's rights to positions. And it is this, I believe, that makes preferential treatment appear so morally odious. To violate rights is generally seen to be (correctly) a very serious matter and to allow rights to be overridden, particularly for consequential reasons, seems to strike at the heart of a moral idea that is fundamental to our entire moral code. (If these rights are tradable, then what will be the next to go in the pursuit of some other 'dubious' social goal?)

None of this is to argue against preferential treatment *per se* (or, indeed, for it); it is, rather, a matter of establishing the case that the moral stakes are high when we decide on the standing of the practice. The anodyne language in which we often speak of preferential treatment (which is similar to that which we use for affirmative action) tends to disguise the fact that we may be talking about a very important moral concept. But then we must once more enter the caveat that all this depends on the ability of the merit principle to bestow rights to positions.

In order that we can make our arguments apply to most of the areas in which affirmative action and preferential treatment are used, we have briefly to mention two additions to (or possibly variants of) the merit principle. We have already seen that a contentious use of both practices is in the protection of affirmative action gains during lay-offs of employees. Small-scale lay-offs when employees are genuinely redundant may not be so problematical. The difficulty arises when whole groups of workers have to be 'lost' and decisions made about which ones when the question of particular skills redundancy does not arise. In the absence of other more defensible criteria, the most usual practice (particularly in unionised establishments where the principle has been negotiated) is that of seniority or 'last-in-first-out'. If minority employees, taken on under affirmative action programmes, are disproportionately represented among recent hires then they will be most at risk of being laid off under a seniority system. What then, if, in order to protect these minority gains, more senior white employees are layed off in their stead? Is violation of the seniority principle as morally unscrupulous as violation of the merit principle appears to be? Is the seniority principle as morally prescriptive as the merit principle appears to be? Certainly, the Supreme Court has been even more protective of seniority than of merit (on the grounds that there are more particularised victims). But conversely, seniority is often no more than a negotiated arrangement with unions. Furthermore, if we wished to hitch seniority to the merit principle, so to give it more moral muscle, we would soon, I think, come unstuck. Is someone more meritorious (in the sense of being the best person for the job) just because they have been doing it for longer? More to the point, does having been in the job for longer give you more right to it than someone more junior? Clearly the question of seniority presents considerable difficulties for our discussion of preference practice. We shall take up these questions again when we consider the 'innocent victims' argument.

The second variant on merit takes us outside the field of employment. It comes in the form of contract set-asides. If a public agency (a city or state for example) sets aside a fixed percentage of public works contracts (or a fixed percentage of the total annual dollar value of all contracts) for minority companies (a percentage that is greater than they have historically received or are likely to receive), it will in all likelihood override the generally accepted rules and criteria for the award of contracts. In other words, it will end up awarding contracts to companies that have not submitted the cheapest or the best value-for-money tender and (white) companies who would have expected to win the contract by the normal rules of the game would be denied it. (The Croson Company thought that by the normal rules it should have won the contract to install new lavatories in Richmond's prison and as plaintiffs in subsequent legal action got the Supreme Court for the first time to consider the matter of lavatory installation – and then deliver a judgement that threw the procedure of contract set-asides into disarray across the country.)

On initial consideration it would appear that to by-pass normal rules and procedures in the award of contracts does not constitute a breach of moral principles in the way that violating the merit principle might. Breaking rules does not strike us as being so serious as breaching moral principles. And if that is the case, then preferential treatment in contract set-asides may be less unacceptable than its use in hiring and promotion. In the next chapter we give further consideration to the merit principle which will raise doubts about its moral apodicity and narrow the acceptability gap between contract set-asides and overriding merit. For the moment, however, we have said enough about the practice of affirmative action and preferential treatment in hiring, promotion, seniority lay-offs and contract set-asides to indicate the ideal-type distinction between the two. The borderline is crossed when practices appear to abrogate some principle or conventional rules of behaviour. The principle abrogated in hiring and promotion appears to be the morally strong one of rights to positions; elsewhere it seems more likely that preferential treatment will breach the 'rules of the game'.

The symbolic incarnation of preference practice is the quota. Debate about affirmative action and preference almost always crystallises around the distinction between goals and quotas, with the former requiring only good faith efforts within the merit principle, the latter falling under the long and infamous shadow of the *numerus clausus* with its requirement to disregard merit to achieve the quota. We have already seen that there is a degree of spuriousness in the goal/quota distinction, with the affirmative action culture often driving the former into the latter. Notwithstanding that, however, there is a strong symbolic and legal content to the quota and it has remained at the centre of the debate in the United States (see, for example, Abram 1986, Belton 1981, Steele 1990b, Cooper 1991, *Congressional Quarterly Researcher* 1991b, Belz 1991) and underpinned President Bush's opposition to the 1990 Civil Rights Act (he took the view that employers would be forced into using quotas in order to avoid disparate impact lawsuits).

ENDS AND MEANS

Do the purposes for which race-conscious policies are pursued affect the morality of preference? In general terms the answer to this must of course be 'yes'. Practices that are pursued in fulfilment of the demands of justice or rights, even when they appear to upset other moral principles, may be justified in a way that they could not be if the purpose was expediency or utility or more general consequence (see Edwards 1987). In practice, however, the debate about the moral standing of affirmative action and preference in the United States (and even more so in the United Kingdom) has been relatively indifferent to the ends being pursued, particularly during the past decade.

We have identified four principal reasons for using race-conscious practices in the United States, three of which apply also in Great Britain. The first is what Goldman (1976) has called the forward-looking purpose but which really incorporates two distinct reasons: racial equity and equality of opportunity. Of the two, equality of opportunity is the more often cited as a justification (or reason) for race-conscious practice (see for example Goldman 1977, Sher 1977, 1987, Fishkin 1987, Fullinwider 1986). Now equality of opportunity is problematic for a number of reasons, as we have already seen, but the question that confronts us here is whether it constitutes a moral value of the kind that justice requires to be met or rather (simply) a utility enhancing rule. Fullinwider has defended equality of opportunity as a sounder basis for affirmative action (at least insofar as it is used in consent decrees) than compensation or restitution, but it remains unclear from his exposition whether he is treating equality of opportunity as morally apodictic or as promoting utility:

> the fact that preferential programs benefit the best qualified blacks or women instead of the most injured constitutes an embarrassment for the compensatory defence, but not for the defence in terms of equal opportunity. If the aim is to reform institutional habits, then it is irrelevant that those whose presence can most effectively accomplish this change are themselves relatively advantaged.

The forward-looking defence does not have to find some special deservingness in the beneficiaries of preference since it *does not view*

them as receiving their benefits by right. They are given preferences
because it serves the larger aim.

(Fullinwider 1986: 184, emphasis added)

Fullinwider has already noted that there is a difficulty in ascribing to
the beneficiaries of a compensatory programme rights to the positions
they have obtained because the *particular* beneficiary may not be
deserving of compensation (and his or her location in that position is
in effect as a proxy for all minorities who as a group deserve compensation). It is not clear, however, why he asserts that beneficiaries of
forward-looking programmes have no rights to positions (or why this
makes preference more defensible). We can surmise three possible
reasons why this might be so. First, equality of opportunity does not in
itself bestow rights. This must logically be true because equal opportunity *per se* bestows nothing; it is only when hitched to selection by merit
that it can be said to promote the desired result that the best person
will get the job. This does not appear to be what Fullinwider has in mind.
Second, it may be asserted that the beneficiary of a preference programme (pursued for whatever reason) has no right to the position
precisely because they have been preferred over someone else better
qualified under existing rules and criteria. For a proponent of affirmative action to argue thus seems to provide fortune with some valuable
hostages. It appears, therefore, that we must take Fullinwider at face
value when he implies that the beneficiaries of equal opportunity
preference programmes are merely instruments for the achievement of
a larger aim. Now if this is the case then either it is inconsistent with
the promotion of equal opportunity or Fullinwider has a different
notion of equal opportunity in mind. The logic of using beneficiaries
simply as ciphers must be that it does not matter who gets the position
(provided it is someone from a minority group). This cannot be
consistent with the promotion of individual equality of opportunity. The
alternative might be that Fullinwider is here talking not of individual
equality of opportunity but equality of opportunity between groups – in
which case the beneficiary becomes not an instrument to the achievement of a larger aim, but (as in compensation) a proxy for all members
of minority groups. But such usage is inconsistent with how he treats
equal opportunity in the rest of his argument. The problem remains,
therefore, of whether preference can be used logically, practically and
morally, to promote equality of opportunity. We shall consider equality
of opportunity and the merit principle in more detail in the next
chapter but, rather than leave this question entirely hanging in the air,
we can mark up two potential ways in which preference may promote
equality in opportunities. First, to the extent that preference practices
involve redefining and broadening what counts as merit (as we have
demonstrated), they can bring more people (and a wider variety of

people) into eligibility and consideration for positions. Second, simply to prefer someone for a job may enhance their further opportunities and fulfil potential that was being frustrated by arbitrary barriers.

'Racial equity' I take to mean establishing minority racial groups across the reward system in the proportions that would obtain in the absence of past (and present) discrimination (see Belton 1981, Fiscus 1992). Seen in this way, racial equity bears some resemblance to arguments from compensation insofar as we may assume that the latter is an attempt to right past wrongs not in order to reinstate the status quo ante (which has no meaning in the context of racial oppression) but rather to effect a sort of Nozickian restitution to the position that minorities would now hold had they not been discriminated against. The purposes are similar and there seems to be no good reason for not attributing to the promotion of racial equity the same moral standing that we do to compensation.

The most extensive treatment of racial equity (though he does not use that term to describe it) is to be found in Fiscus's work on proportionate and disproportionate quotas (Fiscus 1992). Briefly stated, his argument is that if we assume no systematic differences between racial and ethnic groups in intelligence, aptitudes, talents, abilities and so on (and there is, he argues, no reason for assuming otherwise), and given a complete absence of discrimination between races, then logic must dictate that there will be no systematic differences in the distribution of racial groups across the reward system. There just would not have been any processes at work that could have produced any other but this result. (He acknowledges that different *ethnic* groups with varying cultures may make systematically different choices in occupations which may result in non-proportional representation, but argues that is it quite wrong to equate ethnic with racial groups. He does not acknowledge, on the other hand, that disproportionate representation of ethnic groups must *ipso facto* skew the distribution for other groups. Thus, if cultural disposition leads to a concentration of one ethnic group in (say) the medical profession, other groups must be under-represented in this profession compared with their representation in the population as a whole.) Fiscus then uses the argument of proportional representation based on equality at birth to justify the use of 'proportionate quotas' to re-establish the distribution of minorities that should now exist had discrimination not occurred. Thus, if (say) 20 per cent of the population are black then 20 per cent of doctors should be black as should 20 per cent of admissions to medical school (there being no reason in the absence of discrimination and oppression why blacks would *not* be so represented). In this example (it relates to the Davis Medical School at the University of California) 20 per cent of places in medical schools should go to blacks *by right*. But no more; anything above 20 per cent would be an unjustified 'disproportionate quota'. On these grounds (as Fiscus points out) Allan Bakke was not entitled to the place he claimed to have a right to because although his test scores put him among the top 100 per cent of successful white applicants and were higher than those of some of the minority candidates admitted under the Davis programme, he did not score among the top 80 per cent of successful white candidates and was therefore ineligible for one of the 80 per cent of places for which he had an entitlement to compete (see Fiscus 1992: 37–39). In this manner, Fiscus claims he is able to dispense with the 'innocent victim' argument. There is an appealing simplicity to the argument (and it remains one of the best defences of quotas) but it also remains unsettling for reasons that we shall only touch upon here but will take up in more detail in subsequent paragraphs. The disquiet arises from the apparent elision of group and individual rights. A common argument against quotas for compensatory purposes (and echoed in the passage from Fullinwider above) is that they represent a very crude compensatory mechanism in that the minority beneficiaries – especially of programmes such as that at Davis – are unlikely to be amongst the most harmed. Indeed, they are now among the most advantaged of the group. The most harmed will be the least likely to benefit from university entrance programmes. Now our concern is not (at present) with the substance of this argument but rather with the fact that it introduces an intra-group dimension. Compensatory quotas are wrong (so the argument goes) because the *wrong* minority group members benefit. It will be recalled that Fullinwider saw no equivalent problem with equal opportunity quotas because the best qualified minorities would benefit and this was consistent with equality of opportunity.[1] Fiscus likewise disavows compensatory arguments and for broadly similar reasons – that they give rise to intra-group injustices (unharmed blacks benefit to the disadvantage of harmed blacks, and innocent whites pay the costs of compensation to the advantage of guilty whites). He then goes on to commend proportionate quotas (for racial equity) on the grounds that they do not incur the same moral costs. And this is because (presumably) they do not give benefits to the wrong people or, to put it another way, whilst being group practices, they remain sensitive to other morally relevant criteria of distribution – in this case merit. It must follow therefore that the *individual* members of the minority group who do benefit under Fiscus's preference system are the same ones who would have benefited had there never been oppression and discrimination. This, to say the least, is a very heroic assumption. It requires us to believe that over the history of oppression of minority groups the opportunities, life-chances, talents, abilities and so on of each individual minority group member have been suppressed to exactly the same degree. That means uniform oppression with uniform results. And this just is not a plausible assumption. It is asking too much to have us believe that particular and identifiable preference beneficiaries are the same ones who have a right to positions on the basis of primordial merit. (The same must apply of course – though not for the same reasons – to majority beneficiaries of merit.) I believe we must return therefore to the position stated earlier that, morally speaking, there is a close similarity between compensation and equality of opportunity (and now, equity). Just as we cannot assume that compensatory benefits under preference programmes go to the 'right' people, neither can we assume this to be the case under the application of current time-slice merit principles. Either we must say that (for a variety of reasons) it does not matter within the group who benefits from preference programmes or we have to concede that they are poor instruments for distributing intra-group compensation *and* merit rewards. That having been said, it has to be acknowledged that if we are concerned with intra-group desert then in practice equal-opportunity preference will be less damaging to justice than compensatory preference if only because the latter has a tendency to provide benefit in inverse relation to compensatory desert. Both forms of preference however must have a tendency to intra-group injustice.

Philosophical arguments for affirmative action and preferential treatment in America have traditionally revolved around the question of compensation for past harm though as Fullinwider has argued, this has tended to be replaced since the late 1970s by a growing emphasis on diversity and equality of opportunity as reasons for promoting race-conscious practices (Fullinwider 1986). Notwithstanding this shift, however, compensation still infiltrates the debate and almost all Supreme Court opinions in affirmative action and related cases over the past two decades have contained elements (at least) of the compensation argument. Indeed, it seems that no matter how avowedly forward-looking the rationale for affirmative action and preference might be, it is impossible completely to ignore the question of compensatory costs and benefits if only because preference policies will themselves create such beneficiaries and victims whatever the reason for their promotion. Thus, although Fiscus dismisses the compensation-for-past-harm argument as a basis for race-conscious practices, he is forced to devote at least a quarter of a (albeit unfinished) book to a discussion of victims and beneficiaries which turns out to be an inescapable component of compensation (Fiscus 1992).

We shall not rehearse here all the arguments (there are many) about race-conscious practices as a means of effecting compensation or restitution (a different thing) for past harm and violation of rights (useful examples may be found in Bittker 1973, Boxhill 1977, Blackstone and Heslep 1977, Goldman 1976, 1977, Eastland and Bennett 1979, Gross 1978 and Day 1981), because the important issues that such arguments raise find a place in subsequent paragraphs. It is enough to say at this stage that the moral foundation for backward-looking affirmative action and preferential treatment appears prima facie to be a strong one. It is incontrovertible that great harm has been done to some minority groups (and more to some than to others); that the legacy of this harm remains and that justice is not done if the costs of this harm are simply allowed to lie where they fall. Some may argue that the time for compensation has passed, that it was all a long time ago and that we cannot attribute the relatively deprived status of (some) groups today to the continuation of damage done decades ago (see Abram 1986, J.E. O'Neill 1987, Sowell 1990, Steele 1990b). We should not dismiss such arguments too lightly (though in their more simplistic forms they owe much to the pull-themselves-up-by-their-bootlaces school of thinking) because they do at least (or should) direct our minds to the diversity of minority groups and their very different histories in American (and British) society. It is proper that we should remind ourselves that when we talk about compensation for past harm we have, as likely as not, the history of African-Americans in mind. But the programmes we are evaluating apply equally to people of Hispanic origin, to American Indians, to Aleut and to Asians (and to West Indians in both America and Britain). All these groups have suffered very different degrees of harm and now occupy different positions in the reward system (see Hacker 1989, Van Alstyne 1979). The fact that we apply the same compensatory programmes to all of them and group them together for the purposes of goal setting may itself be a measure not only of policy ineptitude but of injustice as well. After all, what sense does it make in compensatory terms preferentially to hire Asians or Hispanics as a way of righting the wrongs done to blacks?

The third broad justification for race-conscious policies, and the most recent, is the promotion of diversity. Though diversity was an issue in *Bakke*, it is really over the past ten years that it has increasingly displaced compensation, equality of opportunity and racial equity as the dominant basis for policy (see Mishkin 1983, Hacker 1989, Carter 1991). The attractiveness of diversity over other rationales is its moral adaptability and the fact that it does not lay claim to what may increasingly look to many people as the specious moral high ground of righting wrongs and promoting justice. As appropriate, diversity can be an end in itself – and a transparently commonsensical one (who after all is going to gainsay that America's rich diversity should be reflected in its factories, offices and major institutions) – or a means to many other valuable ends not the least of which will be the demographic necessity of broadening the labour force base.

In its latter form, diversity is but one example of a broader category of justifications (the fourth type) for race-conscious practices. These we may call broadly consequential arguments.[2] Some may be more particularly utilitarian (see Dworkin 1977a, 1977b, Blackstone 1977, R. O'Neil 1975). The ends to be served by consequence-based, race-conscious policies vary considerably in type but, more importantly for present purposes, they differ also in their relation to the good of relevant minorities. In this respect, some are more morally compelling than others – or at least we might think so. Is not the moral case for group practices different, for example, if they are pursued on the one hand in order to provide more minority doctors, policemen and other professionals better to serve minority communities, and on the other to promote business, or in the hope of defusing the likelihood of civil unrest? The first is at least consistent with the general purpose of group practices – to improve the condition of the affected groups – whereas the latter two subordinate this general purpose to broader and more general ones which may (but also may not) be to the benefit of such groups. It follows from the logic of means and ends, therefore, that if improving the conditions of racial and religious minorities was not functional for increased profitability or defusing civil unrest, it would not be done. Quite simply, it is not an end in itself and to treat the betterment of groups simply as a means to other ends is not a morally compelling reason for action.

More generally speaking, it will almost always be the case, even where affirmative action and preferential treatment are used to improve services to minority communities, that the deontic arguments for these practices will be more morally compelling than teleologic ones. Whilst no policy practices can be entirely blind to consequences, it is reasonable to argue (as do for example Barry, Brandt, Singer and Rawls) that the apodictic demands of justice and rights are more morally compelling than those of consequence even if the consequence is utility maximising (see Barry 1965, 1967, Brandt 1979, Singer 1979, Rawls 1972). Thus, if people have been harmed by culpable agents and have rights to compensation, there are compelling moral grounds for effecting this, and unintended consequences (even if foreseen) must be a subordinate consideration. Likewise, if distributive justice requires distributions in proportion to need (along with other things) and if race-conscious practices provide an effective way of doing this, then this is a more morally compelling argument for their implementation than is general consequence.[3]

THE COSTS OF PREFERENCE

Irrespective of the justifications for race-conscious practices, the practices themselves are relatively invariable. One might expect that practices followed for compensatory purposes would be differently tailored from ones the aims of which were to promote racial equity or to equalise opportunities and that these in turn would differ from those constructed for consequential or utilitarian reasons. This is not the case, as we have seen from earlier examples, and ought in itself to be a cause for concern. Though the costs of preference policies must be weighed against a variety of justifications of varying moral strength, the costs themselves will be fairly common because they derive from common practices.

The most commonly cited cost of preferential policies is that they violate other people's rights to positions under the merit principle or, as we have seen in the case of contract set-asides, entitlement under customary rules. There are, however, a number of antecedent questions that in part give rise to the concern about rights-violations and we shall consider some of these in the remainder of this chapter. We shall also examine the arguments about the innocent victims of preference policies but will hold over the questions of rights to positions until the next chapter because it deserves more extended treatment in the context of equality of opportunity and the merit principle.

The signal characteristic of both affirmative action and preferential treatment practices that we identified in an early chapter is that they are group practices and that the groups at their focus are morally arbitrarily defined. The groups may be (usually are) identified because of some morally relevant characteristic held in common by some, or all, members (rights to compensation, greater needs and so on) but the beneficiaries themselves are identified (in the present context) by characteristics of race or ethnicity. It is this signal characteristic that gives rise to moral difficulties and from which stem most of the perceived or real costs of such policies. We shall consider the following components of the morally arbitrary group problem: groups rights versus individual rights; the selection of affected groups; whether individual beneficiaries of preference can be proxies for whole groups; and the nature of the injury suffered by groups.

Group rights and individual rights

If it can be established that a morally arbitrary group has rights *qua* group then it necessarily follows that the group has moral standing. (The reverse is not the case; a group may have moral standing of some kind without that extending to having rights.) Do group rights exist, and if they do, how do they come about?

Rights-talk is notoriously permissive and has in consequence lost some of its value. Over the past two decades a number of groups have claimed for themselves rights which are not distinguishable rights at all. Gay rights, lesbian rights, women's rights are of dubious standing. Homosexuals have no different rights than heterosexuals; the only basis upon which homosexuals as a group may claim rights is by a showing of harm done that justifies a right to compensation. Many would argue precisely this but the result has tended to be a degree of 'oppression inflation' or 'oppression fatigue'; and the result of this is that we end up taking less seriously than we should the condition of seriously deprived groups. Before we can establish whether a particular group has a group right to something, we must see whether and how group rights exist at all and, equally importantly, whether they can coexist with individual rights.

What might morally arbitrary groups in theory have a right to? As material principles of justice, harm and need may establish prima-facie rights to compensation and to having needs met. In addition, we can say that whilst there can be no presumption of equality *per se* (between people or groups), there is a right to be treated as equals (see Dworkin 1977a: Chapter 9) or to equal consideration. And from a right to equal consideration it is possible to derive a right to equality of opportunity if we assume (as appears reasonable) that a right to equal consideration must entail discounting or compensating for needs or disadvantages that arbitrarily restrict people from being counted as equals. We are not being treated as equals, in other words, if unnecessary and arbitrary handicaps are allowed to count against us (see Edwards 1993).

If we assume then that such rights as compensatory, need, treatment as equals and equality of opportunity do exist, how do groups (as opposed to individuals) acquire them? Broadly speaking the answer must be 'in the same manner in which groups may attain moral standing' – that is, by association with a morally relevant criterion. A high correlation between group membership and past harm or present levels of need (so this argument would go) would establish prima-facie rights to *group* compensation and to resources to meet needs. Such a derivation must be subject to the same qualifications that we noted earlier in respect of establishing moral standing in general, but where rights are concerned we are faced with some new dilemmas because if such things as group rights exist, they may (and almost certainly will) conflict with individual rights. Before we comment further on this, however, it is worth noting some more general questions raised by the notion of group rights.

If we assume (because of perfect correlation with a morally relevant factor or for some other compelling reason) that a morally arbitrary group does have *group* rights that are distinguishable from the rights that individual members have (as they must be if the concept is to have any meaning), what is the *nature* of these rights? Just what does it mean to say that a morally arbitrary group has rights? And what (or who) *is* it that holds the right? (Do racial groups, for example, have some sort of *corporate* identity?) Does each and every member of the group hold the right in virtue of being a member of the group or is it the case, as Bayles has argued, that 'since the obligation [to compensate] is to the group, no specific individual has a right to reparation' (Bayles 1973b: 183)?

And if Bayles is correct, does this mean that identifiable individual beneficiaries of preferential treatment based on group rights have no rights to the jobs or positions they have thereby gained? The consequences of this (if true) for the beneficiaries of preference policies are unsettling to say the least.

The 'cleanest' example of fulfilling a group right (to compensation) would be that of reparation payments to all black people as proposed in the Black Manifesto in 1969 (see Bittker 1973, Fullinwider 1980: 25ff.) but even this, though based on a per capita sum, was to have been used for collective purposes and would therefore have produced variable individual benefit. Affirmative action and preferential treatment do not present even this relative degree of neatness however. We shall consider two arguments that at the minimum qualify the idea of group rights. The first starts from the fact that a justification from association with morally relevant factors (need, harm) relies upon an association between the relevant variable on the one hand and group membership on the other, among *individual* class members. Thus, the idea of a *group* injury (for example) calling forth a *group* right to compensation is ultimately dependent on the degree of association between morally relevant and morally arbitrary factors among *individual* members of the group. So long as collective rights are based on association at the individual level, therefore, it is hard to sustain the view that they are different from, and independent of, individual rights. Probably the most cogent reasoning to circumvent this difficulty is to argue that the association between morally relevant and arbitrary criteria is not one between individual *rights* to compensation for harm and group membership but more simply between harm suffered and group membership. The group as a whole has suffered more harm than other groups and this, quite irrespective of any individual rights involved, gives rise to the group right. There is, I believe, sufficient substance in this argument at least to allow us to proceed to the next hurdle. This concerns the questions, in who (or what) does a group right reside, if it exists, and who or what is the proper beneficiary of action taken to fulfil it? These questions are brought into sharper focus by the implementation of preference policies. We have noted before that the individual beneficiaries of preference (and affirmative action) practices are quixotically chosen. They are in effect those minority group members who are in the right place at the right time and have the appropriate qualifications – or at least not much below them (see Hoffman 1977). They have benefited because a *group* right has been assumed and they have been thrown up by arbitrary circumstances as its fortunate beneficiaries. Others (most others) in the group have not benefited from preference practices. By what justifiable means then has the group right settled on this arbitrarily selected sub-set and provided a conduit for benefits to them (and not to others)? Do these particular individuals have rights (individual rights) in virtue of there being a group right? And if they do, why do *they* have this particular right when it is denied to other members of the group by happenstance or a greater deprivation that has prevented them from being in a position from which they could benefit from preferential university entry or preferential access to better jobs? It seems that if we are to accept the idea of group rights we must accept that they will necessarily be blind to individual rights and may even act in opposition to them.

The only plausible counter to this rather damaging account of group rights is once again to argue that these particular beneficiaries have gained *only* because there is a group right and the group right to compensation or need-meeting is fulfilled by benefit to *any* member of the group who in this sense will be a proxy for all other members. The beneficiaries, in other words, are not having an individual right fulfilled because they do not have individual rights and thus there can be no conflict between group and individual rights. But such a counter-argument is itself flawed – and probably fatally so. In essence, it can mean one of two things. Either it means that group rights do not bestow individual rights but that nonetheless quite separate and independent individual rights remain, or that where group rights are established, individual rights cease to exist. The latter is implausible; even if individuals could trade away their individual rights for a group right, it is unlikely that they would do so, particularly if the subsequent beneficiaries were to be chosen quixotically. The former version is self-defeating. Even if the beneficiaries are only proxies, ciphers, embodiments of the whole group, they have still obtained a benefit (job, university place, etc.) that probably ought to have gone to another member of the same group on the basis of individual right.[4]

What groups?

If affirmative action and preference policies create injustices between individuals, neither do they appear to discriminate fairly between groups. Indeed, as we have seen from the examples in earlier chapters, these practices are remarkably indiscriminate with respect to beneficiary groups in both Great Britain and the United States. This promiscuity operates at two levels. First, as between different racial and ethnic groups and second between them and other groups such as the disabled, homosexuals and women. Similar practices are usually employed in respect of all these groups irrespective of the relative degrees of harm they have suffered or the needs they have (as, for example, in *Richmond v. Croson*). (And the disabled do not constitute a morally arbitrary group – they have additional needs by definition – and the moral dilemmas of affirmative action and preference do not apply to them.) Sometimes (as in the SA Company – see Chapter 6) goals are set within which women and racial minorities are interchangeable. And in almost all cases, goals are set for all racial minorities combined (even though prior analyses are broken down by discrete group).

The point need not be laboured. There are very few (if any) groups in either Britain or the United States that have even similar histories of oppression and discrimination. Almost all groups differ in the progress they have made and are making. There is little reason why Asians in America ('Chinese' Asians as opposed to Indian sub-continent Asians in Great Britain) should remain a protected group (Hacker 1989, Kirp and Weston 1987: 244–45). Jews long ago ceased to hold this status. West Indian Americans are not afforded a status separate from that of African-Americans yet their pattern of progress is very different. It might not matter for the purpose of race-conscious practice that whilst 'African-American' is a racial classification, 'Hispanic', 'Chicano' and 'Latino' represent ethnic groups, but as Skerry points out (in an article admittedly critical of some affirmative action practice) most of the 600,000 or so legal immigrants to the United States, and almost all of the 100,000 to 300,000 illegal immigrants in 1989 (the average annual rate since the Immigration Reform and Control Act of 1986), were of Hispanic origin. These immigrants, he claims, will enter the country and immediately be able to adopt the status of an oppressed group and be eligible for benefit from preference policies (Skerry 1989). One does not have to agree with the sentiments to see the point. *Compared with African-Americans*, Hispanics are recent arrivals. Should they be afforded the same status as blacks in preference programmes? (And conversely, if they should not, should they be afforded the same status with whites as 'oppressors'?)

In some areas of affirmative action and preference, some of this will not matter, given relatively high degrees of residential segregation. If the labour draw area is predominantly black, the programmes, if successful, will pull in blacks even if the goal relates to 'all minorities'. But what if the draw area is mixed (black, Hispanic, Asian) and the programme pulls in predominantly Asian candidates and they fill the goal? There seems no good reason now for not disaggregating goals and setting targets for each protected group where this is appropriate in the light of availability data.

The practice of goal disaggregation is in fact happening informally on a fairly wide scale already. It has yet to become widespread as a formal practice however. Where it has happened, it has been assisted I believe by the emergence of 'diversity' and the decline of 'compensation' as the driving force of race-conscious programmes. The compensation argument remained palatable so long as it dealt in generalities. To subject it to fine tuning by requiring separate but proportionately equal goals for each and every group would expose it to an indefensible critique. Serious (and ultimately embarrassing) efforts would have to be made to calculate the relative harms suffered by each group and then to tailor remedial programmes accordingly. It just would not work. Diversity, on the other hand, *requires* that a mix of groups be created and enables this to be done without the complexity of worrying about history.

Fortuitous beneficiaries and innocent victims

No other aspect of preference practice raises such obvious moral dilemmas as the question of whether the beneficiaries and losers get their just deserts. It emerges most frequently as the 'innocent victim' argument which deals with one side of the equation, but the other side which we might call 'fortuitous beneficiaries' has also exercised the Supreme Court on a number of occasions. Many of the arguments on each side of the equation complement each other but they are more comprehensible if kept separate. We shall consider first concerns about 'innocent victims'.

Unnecessary confusion has sometimes arisen from a failure to separate two levels of argument about the victims[5] and beneficiaries of affirmative action and preference. There will be beneficiaries and losers of affirmative action and preference (as of many other public and private practices) whatever the reason for pursuing those practices. The mechanics of the process will dictate this. And if the practices are used to promote diversity or for other consequential reasons, then it may not matter, as we have noted already, *who* (which individuals) the beneficiaries are. (It may still matter, however, who bears the costs.) The moral costs and benefits of practices used in this way have to be weighed against relatively diffuse criteria (such as whether the end to be achieved justifies the costs to the losers; whether the appointment of *any* minority group member (sufficiently qualified) will serve equally to produce the desired end, and so on). When, however, preference practice is used for the purposes of compensation, the criteria for evaluation are both more precise and narrow. *If* race-conscious practices are used explicitly for compensatory purposes then the test of their validity and effectiveness will be whether the right people pay the costs. And this must be so even if the 'right people' in each case are all (or all existing) members of a class. It is ironic, therefore, in the light of what we have said earlier about the shift in the justification for race-conscious policies from compensation to the promotion of diversity and for other consequential reasons, that almost all of the debate in America about the victims and beneficiaries of these policies has been, and continues to be, formulated within the context of compensation for past harm or wrongs.

One of the major concerns of the Supreme Court, for example, when it has considered affirmative action and related cases, has been with the distribution of the burdens and benefits of compensatory practice. One of the reasons why the Court found Kaiser Aluminum's Grammercy plan not to violate Title VII of the Civil Rights Act was that it did not 'unnecessarily trammel the interests of the white employees' (*United Steelworkers v. Weber* 1979). In both *Stotts* and *Wygant*, which involved seniority in lay-offs and the threat that this posed for affirmative action gains, the Court found support for the seniority system in part (and in both cases) because overriding seniority to protect minority gains would involve costs falling on identifiable white 'innocent employees' (*Firefighters Local Union No. 1785 v. Stotts* 1984). In *Wygant*,[6] Justice Powell made a clear distinction between affirmative action hiring practices and affirmative action in lay-offs: 'Denial of a future employment opportunity is not as intrusive as loss of an existing job. While hiring goals impose a diffuse burden ... layoffs impose the entire burden of achieving racial equality on *particular individuals* ...' (*Wygant v. Jackson Board of Education* 1986). A decade earlier than *Wygant*, however, the Court had taken a rather different view of the questions of benefits and costs. *Franks v. Bowman Transportation Co.* concerned the award of retroactive seniority to black employees who had been the victims of past discrimination. The award resulted in a relative loss of seniority for some (identifiable) white employees. The Supreme Court upheld the award and rejected the argument that it deprived white employees of seniority rights. The amelioration of 'the effects of past racial discrimination [is] a national policy objective of the highest priority', the Court argued, and as such, the burden of correcting it should be shared by both black and white employees (*Franks v. Bowman Transportation Co.* 1976). Of course, it is necessary to read Supreme Court decisions in the light of who its constituent members are at any given time, but as an *institution* it has clearly not been able to pass down an incontrovertibly unambiguous message on the harms and benefits of preference.

Who bears the costs of preference (or who you think ought to) will, of course, depend in large measure on how the 'preferred' groups have been defined. It has become customary to use white males as the quintessential victims[7] but this rests only on the current orthodoxy that only white males have been responsible for past oppression (and continue to be). Since this is a highly unempirical assertion, I shall refer to the alleged victims of preference as whites except when discussing particular references to 'white males'. Any other group may be inserted as desired to reflect the reader's chosen pecking order of preference.

The complaint about preference policies when they are used for compensatory purposes is that they are a very poor mechanism for achieving this. The reason, as we have seen, is the simple one that the costs of preference fall serendipitously on those whites who do not get the job or the promotion or the university place that they would have got had a minority candidate not been preferred.[8] The principle of compensation requires that only those who have been wronged, or harmed, or both, should receive compensation, and only those 'guilty' of harm-doing or wrong-doing should pay the costs of compensation. It further requires (ideally) that compensation should be in proportion to the harm suffered and the costs be in proportion to the harm inflicted (see Fullinwider 1986: 174–79). Preference policies, it is argued, do none of these things (see Gross 1977, Sher 1977, Nagel 1977, Goldman 1979: Chapter 3, Greene 1977). Such policies function through the job market and other selection procedures;[9] it is no part of them to seek out present and past harm-doers and deprive *them* of a position. There is no way of telling whether the white victim is a harm-doer. We may in consequence be loading the costs of compensation on the innocent victim.

Now what is it that makes the white person who does not get the position a 'victim'? Had she failed to get the position in 'fair competition'[10] (i.e. someone better qualified than her was appointed) we would not call her a victim. Because a woman from a racial minority group who is less qualified for the job on the customary criteria gets it, she (the white woman) becomes a victim. Why is this? It is because we think (intuitively) that as the best qualified candidate she has a reasonable expectation or an entitlement or a right to the position. And we think this because those are the rules of the game or what in more elevated parlance is called the merit principle. This is but the sketchiest outline of the idea of rights to positions (we discuss in the next chapter why it is faulty) but it provides sufficient on which to hang a counter-argument (and a defence of preference).

The counter to the 'victims' argument is simply that they are not victims because they had no rights or entitlements to the positions, failure to achieve which has given them victim status. *Why* they had no such rights comes in a variety of forms. The two most often cited are that in the absence of the oppression of, and discrimination against, minorities, they (the whites) might not have been in the position they now are. Their present relatively elevated position has been gained on the backs of oppressed minorities. They are where they are now because of the harm they have done to others (see Thomson 1986, Bittker 1973). The variant of this is that the institutions to which they have just failed to gain entry are creations of a white society that in the past has drawn up the rules of the game in such a way as to benefit whites. On either variant it may then be argued that although *current* losers from preference programmes may not themselves be guilty of having caused harm to, or wronged, minorities, they are nonetheless *beneficiaries* of that harm. And this must apply to *all* whites (or all white males, etc.). This is a view that has been cogently put by Judith Jarvis Thomson:

the costs are imposed [in this analysis] on the young white male applicants who are turned away. And so it should be noticed that it is not entirely inappropriate that those applicants should pay the costs. No doubt few, if any, have themselves, individually, done any wrongs to blacks and women. But they have profited from the wrongs the community did.

(Thomson 1986: 152)

Now this, it seems to me, is a crucial issue, because it is over this ground that the arguments for and against preference must engage. If (to trespass briefly on the subject matter of the next chapter) we can argue that the merit principle is not pure enough to grant rights to positions, then an important hurdle is removed from the path towards accepting preferential treatment. But there remains the not inconsiderable inconvenience that some people will be deprived of positions which they might have had a reasonable expectation (but not a right) of obtaining under the customary (even if impure) rules for hiring, promoting and appointing. If, then, Thomson is correct in her assertion that it is not inappropriate for these same people to bear these costs (unfulfilled expectations) because they have benefited from past wrongs then this second hurdle is also removed and the way seems clearer to approving the moral standing of preference.

Thomson's assertion, however, is far from incontestable because it shifts the ground upon which the notion of liability rests and it does so in two ways. First, customary thinking (in tort law for example) requires that for guilt, and thus potential liability for remedy, to be established, some immediate or proximate causal connection must be established between the harm done and the alleged harm-doer. This need not be (and under the Griggs Doctrine is not) intentional causation; it simply requires that action or inaction on the part of one agent is causally connected to harm to another, whether intended or not (see Belton 1981: 535, Fullinwider 1980: Chapter 2, Alexander 1990). This requirement for demonstrating liability to bear the cost of remedy is not met in Thomson's example. There is no suggestion that the young white males she cites have caused harm – indeed she acknowledges quite the opposite (Thomson 1986: 152). There is little ground upon which their liability to remedy (which in this case represents not getting a job or position) can be based in terms of causation of harm.

White males' liability to pay the costs of remedy in Thomson's arguments then requires another shift in ground. Instead of guilt and liability being made dependent on *causing* harm, it is made to derive from *receiving benefit* from someone else's wrong-doing (Thomson 1986: 152, Boxhill 1977: 276–77, Fullinwider 1980: Chapter 2). Boxhill has noted for example:

> The argument under consideration simply does not depend on or imply the claim that white people are culpable or blameable; the argument is that merely by being white, an individual receives benefits to which others have at least partial rights. In such cases, whatever one's choice or moral culpability, reparation must be made.
>
> (Boxhill 1977: 276–77)[11]

Now, as Fullinwider observes, the shift from guilt by causation to guilt by benefiting is a fairly radical one if we are intending to load the costs of compensation or reparation on the guilty (see Fullinwider 1986: 175). Just as there are degrees of guilt, so there are degrees of benefiting. We may wish to call guilty an accomplice who knowingly benefits from a crime that he or she knows about. But what of unwitting beneficiaries? Certainly they have no entitlement to the benefit derived from harm to others, by others, but if they are unaware that the benefit is so derived would we wish to count them as guilty as the knowing accomplice? Intuition would argue otherwise. This defence falls, however, if it is argued (as Boxhill does) that the facts of history are too well known for any white (or white male) to claim ignorance of the fact that the benefit he has gained might, in the absence of past wrong-doing and harm, have belonged to someone of another racial group.

A more telling argument against guilt by benefit, particularly when whole groups are concerned, lies in the nature of the cost to be borne and its distribution among those liable. How can a white person avoid complicity in the harm-doing? (We must assume that avoiding complicity is a better and more noble course of action than taking the benefit in the knowledge that it has been ill-gained.) Are all white (males) guilty or only those who gain or already hold positions that ought rightfully to be held by minority group members? If all white (males) are guilty, does that mean that none of them should now be in the positions they hold? Surely this cannot be what is intended. But if not this, then *which* white (male) position holders and gainers should not by rights be where they are? These questions must be posed because they are the logical extension of guilt-by-benefit and they point up, because of their unanswerability, the fatal flaws in the argument. How then can (let us say) a white male avoid complicity? Let us assume that he wishes to apply for a position but wishes to avoid compounding past harm by accepting a job that would be ill-gained. The only way in which his 'innocence' can be established (other than by not applying) would be on a showing that despite affirmative action and preference, no minority group applicant was more entitled to the position even when entitlement was measured on a range of criteria that allowed 'race' to count. In the absence of such a showing, his appointment to the position makes him, prima facie at least, guilty by benefit. His innocence or guilt therefore are quite outwith his power to change; he is deprived of moral choice and stripped of moral autonomy. If it is not in people's power, therefore, to do good by denying unfair benefit, is it not a strange moral argument that insists that they are guilty?

The flaws in the guilt-by-benefit argument have arisen, I believe, because it has been articulated almost entirely in the context of affirmative action and preference – and thus in respect of hiring, promotion and lay-offs. But if it applies to these it must apply equally to *all* jobs and positions. If the argument is true then it just is not good enough for Thomson to argue that 'it is not inappropriate that those [white male] applicants should pay the costs'. It is quite inappropriate because the guilt lies with all white males – as much with those who have been in post for forty years as with new labour market entrants. I believe that the context of preference policies has made an implausible argument look more plausible than it is.

There is a way around this difficulty if we wish to pursue a defence of preferential treatment. It comes in the form of the *numerus clausus* of which Fiscus's proportionate quotas seem to be a version when taken to their logical conclusion. Thus, if we assume that all 'groups' should be represented in all occupations and statuses in the same proportions in which they are found in the 'relevant' population, then we may say that members of any given group have a right to compete only for that proportion of positions appropriate to their group. Thus, if whites make up 60 per cent of the relevant population, they have a right only to 60 per cent of positions, jobs and statuses and white people are only entitled to compete for these. The 40 per cent 'belonging' to other groups will not be available and this will obviate any danger of whites gaining positions which ought to go to members of other groups. The possibility of guilt-by-benefit disappears.

We shall not pursue this line of reasoning in any detail because *numerus clausus* laws are not on any agenda: their history has been one of oppression and repression, not of equity and justice. We should not, however, dismiss Fiscus's notion of proportionate quotas too lightly because this, very approximately, is what many current goals and quotas in Britain and the United States are based upon. Unfortunately, adequate ground-rules for the implementation of quotas have never been articulated. Quotas in use, as we have seen, are immensely crude instruments. Proper ground-rules would need to take account of the following as yet unresolved difficulties. Are all racial, ethnic, gender, religious, etc. groups to be taken into account? If so, there is no basis for arguing (as Fiscus acknowledges) that equality-at-birth must lead to equal representation so far as ethnic and other culturally distinctive groups are concerned. Second, if all such groups are to be counted (and there seems no reason why they should not) then the number of potential proportions into which all jobs, statuses and occupations are to be divided becomes impressive (divide each racial/ethnic/religious group into two sexes for a start). The logistics begin to look impressive too. Third, if each group may compete only for that proportion of positions for which it is entitled[12] this will seriously curtail the opportunities open to members of some groups (female Aleut for example). Fourth, are cross-group flows to be allowed or must positions remain vacant in the event of there being no minimally qualified group member available? Proportionate quotas may be a way around the guilt-by-benefit (or its mirror image, the innocent victim) problem but there would be a high price to pay in other directions it seems.

So far in this section we have been concerned with arguments that derive from the conception of affirmative action and preference as compensation for harm and wrong-doing. What are we to make of the 'innocent victims' question when these practices are in pursuit of diversity, utility or general consequence? Two prefatory points need to be made. First, it ought to depend on the nature of the end being pursued. Some ends will be more justificatory of preference than others. Second, with few exceptions the question of the nature of the ends has been fudged. Universities in America habitually prefer minorities and women in ways that we have shown and this on the grounds of diversity. Yet nowhere is there to be found a cogent argument that diversity justifies not appointing the 'best qualified person'.

Let us then take two types of consequence: the production of more minority doctors better to serve minority communities; and second, diversity. How do these justify preference, and what implications do they have for the innocent victims argument? There are two lines of approach. The first is to accept that the merit principle or the rights to positions of the best qualified do indeed bestow rights and then to argue that what is at issue is the justifiability of overriding these rights in order to achieve some other end. The second is to question the status of the merit principle and the content of merit either to establish that one component of merit may indeed be 'ability to serve some other end' (policing minority areas), or that the true nature of merit is not such as to bestow rights so that the *prima-facie* difficult problem of appearing to sacrifice rights for consequence is rendered otiose. The first approach is the less defensible. To allow rights to be trammelled for the sake of some other end is something we do not accede to lightly and then (usually) only in times of turbulence and for ends that can command general acceptance as constituting 'the common good'. The second approach is more likely to provide a defence of preference when used for consequential reasons. Indeed, the redefinition of merit to include race or ethnic status as a merit value to be taken into account in allocating positions has already become a *de facto* preference practice as we have seen. Thus, if 'diversity' is considered to be an important component for an organisation, something to be cherished or 'celebrated', then being a member of an under-represented group becomes a factor in selection. Or if proper policing of minority communities is highly valued and requires minority policemen and -women to do it, then being a minority group member becomes a merit value in candidates.

Do these arguments overcome any concern for the 'innocent victim'? To answer this head-on, we must put on one side any qualifications we might have about the value of diversity and whether minority professionals *are* necessary for, or better at, servicing minority communities. A defence of preference against the innocent victim charge would then be that a white candidate who failed to gain a position would have done so simply because a minority candidate was better qualified to do the job. He or she would have been ruled out not because of preference for a minority candidate, but simply on the application of the (new) merit principle. There just would be no innocent victims.[13]

The flaw in this defence is easy to see – but quickly runs into difficulties itself. It is that shifting the content of merit to allow more minority candidates to be chosen and to allow *all* candidates to be chosen on merit does not disguise the fact that one component of merit now becomes a factor which everyone *cannot* compete on. It may be a fiction but the sentiment behind equality of individual opportunity is that everyone has an equal ability to compete and an equal opportunity to win. That ceases to be the case if one ineluctable characteristic of an individual disqualifies him or her from the competition. It is a process that in other contexts is called negative discrimination. The difficulty with *this* argument is that one of the most important components of 'traditional' merit – intelligence – also carries a degree of ineluctability.

We turn now to look at the reverse image – the beneficiaries of affirmative action and preference. Do minority gainers from preference policies have some sort of right to the positions they acquire or are they 'fortuitous beneficiaries'? Much of the argument that is relevant here has already been covered and much, as we noted earlier, is a mirror image of the arguments outlined in preceding paragraphs. It will only be necessary to summarise the main points of the debate.

As with other aspects of affirmative action and preference, the Supreme Court has often provided the bones that others have contended over. And as with 'innocent victims' the messages it has sent have not been uncontradictory. The plaintiffs in *Teamsters* used disparate treatment theory (as opposed to disparate impact) to argue that blacks had been discriminated against in promotion and transfer to better jobs. The district court, on a finding of discrimination, ordered the company to give retroactive seniority to the *identifiable* victims. The court of appeals subsequently widened the remedy to include blacks who could not be shown to have suffered specific harm. The Supreme Court then reversed this finding holding that while Title VII enabled a class of people to be used for the purposes of establishing liability, it required, when used for remedial purposes, that only individuals and not a whole class be the subject. Title VII, in other words, only allows remedy for identified victims (Belton 1981, *Teamsters v. United States* 1977). This argument was reaffirmed seven years later by Justice White in *Stotts*. The purpose of Section 706(g) of Title VII, he said, was to provide make-whole relief *only* to the actual victims of illegal discrimination. Two years after Justice White's assertion, Justices Brennan, Marshall, Blackman and Stevens were claiming the opposite in *Local 28*. Section 706(g), they claimed, 'generally does *not* prohibit affirmative race-conscious orders benefiting persons not identifiable as actual victims' (*Local 28 Sheet Metal Workers v. Equal Employment Opportunity Commission* 1986, as cited in Cathcart, Burcham and Sulds 1990: 6). Then, later that same year, the same Justices, joined by Powell and O'Connor, qualified this finding by distinguishing between the intent of Section 706(g) when used in the context of a consent degree as opposed to a court-ordered remedy. Only in the former case would Title VII permit benefits to non-victims (*Local 93 Firefighters v. Cleveland* 1986).

The question of rightful beneficiaries of race-conscious programmes (and the constitutional and statutory standing of such programmes) came increasingly to focus, so far as the Supreme Court was concerned, on how tailored the remedies were to effect compensation for those who had been harmed and only them. Justice Sandra Day O'Connor became the most persistent on this theme. She had already signalled in *Wygant*, joining in a plurality opinion with Justice Powell, that the Equal Protection Clause, whilst not requiring proven employment discrimination in order to sanction racial preference, would require a 'firm basis' for showing that affirmative action was the appropriate remedy (*Wygant v. Jackson Board of Education* 1986). The following year, this time in dissent (joined by Rehnquist and Scalia), Justice O'Connor argued that the 50 per cent black quota for promotions to corporal among Alabama state troopers imposed by the District Court in 1983 was prohibited by the Equal Protection Clause because it was not a 'narrowly tailored' remedy for the problem. (The District Court had imposed the 50 per cent quota – subject to the availability of qualified black candidates – in the face of continued recalcitrance and for a limited period only in order to accelerate the attainment of proportional representation of 25 per cent[14] (*United States v. Paradise*) 1987). The next time that the question of tailored remedies was before the Court, Justice O'Connor was writing for the majority when it struck down Richmond's set-aside programme for minority business enterprises upon which we have already commented. Strict scrutiny was again at issue (see Note 14) but so was the nature of the remedy in relation to the alleged problem. The set-aside of 30 per cent, Justice O'Connor argued, was not a narrowly tailored relief simply because many enterprises could benefit from it that had not and could not possibly have suffered harm from Richmond's past history of discrimination. This was the case, so the court somewhat disingenuously argued, because set-aside contracts would be open to any minority enterprise anywhere in the United States. Preference could thereby be given for a construction contract in Richmond, Virginia, to an Hispanic company in Los Angeles or an Aleut company in Seattle (*City of Richmond v. J.A. Croson* 1989).

As in the matter of victims, therefore, the Supreme Court has not always been consistent in judgements about remedies when these must be assessed in the light of the Equal Protection Clause and strict scrutiny. Pragmatically speaking, the question is really one about how finely tailored a remedial practice should be to compensate or restitute for a harm or wrong-doing. Unfortunately, that does not take us very far unless we can agree on the parameters of the wrong (or the harm – which may be quite different). By 1989 the Supreme Court was clearly adopting a ring-fenced view of wrong. The wrong that Richmond's set-aside was to remedy was the wrong that Richmond city administration has perpetrated, not wrong to blacks or even wrong to blacks in Richmond. And this was all of a piece with the Court's other concern aired in *Croson*, *Ward's Cove* and *Wygant* – that 'general societal dis-crimination' was not enough to warrant remedial programmes. The beneficiaries of such programmes must be the victims of identifiable discriminatory practices by identified institutions. Of course, if the wrong or harm are sufficiently precisely defined and the remedy appropriately tailored, then we are back with compensation to identi-fied harmed individuals and group compensation is ruled out. But that way, as we know, very little compensation is paid and the great majority of those who have been wronged because of a group characteristic go unrecompensed.

Whilst not always going this far, the Supreme Court has increasingly in recent years been exercised by a concern that remedial group practices *should* benefit people who have suffered a manifest harm and do not extend their benefits to those who are unlikely to have been harmed by an identified practice. To this extent, therefore, the Court has *de facto* ruled out a conception of harm and benefit that sees *all* blacks (or all minorities) to have been wronged or harmed.

Now, so long as race-conscious practice is seen in the context of compensation for harm or wrong (the question of the appropriateness of the beneficiaries does not arise to the same extent if diversity or utility is being pursued), then a great deal hinges on whether such programmes are justified as (at least some) recompense for harm or wrong to all members of a group and that the actual beneficiaries have a right to benefit in virtue of being members of the group (which in this case can be the *only* justification for *them* benefiting), or whether they are only appropriate for correcting present (and some past) wrongs to the people who suffered those wrongs. For those who hold to the view that not all living members of minority racial and ethnic groups have been wronged and/or harmed, there is a strong possibility that some at least of the beneficiaries of affirmative action and preference will receive gain to which they are not entitled under a principle of compensation. For those, on the other hand, who think that wrong and harm have passed down the generations, there cannot be undeserving beneficiaries of preference policies. Or so it would seem. But a justification of affirmative action and preference based in whole-group, intergenerational wrong and harm is not unproblematical. Three considerations must be satisfied before we can say with certainty that such practices meet the demands of compensation. Two of these relate to the quixotic way in which beneficiaries of preference are chosen; the third is a more general point about what is being compensated for.

The first consideration concerns the substitutability in compensation of members of one minority group for another. We have seen that the mechanics of affirmative action are relatively crude; goals will usually be set to include members of all protected groups so that in practice a policy designed to correct an under-representation of blacks (resulting from past harm) may do so by preferentially hiring or promoting Hispanics or members of any other group. Now even if we acknowledge, along with advocates of race-conscious policies, that *all* protected groups have been wronged, it stretches credulity, as we have already noted, to say that they have all been wronged in the same way, to the same degree and to the same extent. Though the finding of the Supreme Court in *Richmond v. Croson* was mischievous, some reservations about the substitutability of beneficiaries must surely be in order.

The second concern is similar but centres around substitutability within groups and is in effect another perspective on what we have already had to say about group rights and individual rights. If Boxhill is correct and recompense is owed to all minority group members[15] *qua* members then it appears to matter little *which* members are benefited. They are in effect representatives of the entire group. But in order to maintain this stance, it is necessary to remain blind to the intra-group distribution of harm and recompense and to the requirements of a simple theory of compensation. As Fullinwider notes, a simple model of compensation requires that 'we make good the victim's loss' (Fullinwider 1986: 178) and unless we hold to the view that the harm has been done to the whole group *and indivisibly so*, this must require different levels of benefit for different levels of harm. In other words, compensation must be proportional to harm or wrong. This is not a result that affirmative action and preference achieve.

There is, it must be acknowledged, a risk in arguing that harm has been unequally distributed among (say) all African-Americans, of failing to appreciate the real extent of the wrongs and harms due to the group as a whole. There is an even greater risk of being accused of so doing. So, it must be said that there is no incompatibility between an assertion that all members of a group have been harmed and that this harm has been unequally distributed. It is the assertion that all blacks have been harmed indivisibly that fails to command credibility. The problem remains, therefore, that affirmative action and preference practices do not meet the requirements of a simple model of compensation. Beneficiaries cannot be chosen according to the degree of harm they have suffered and compensation cannot be proportional to harm. Indeed, as others have argued (Fullinwider 1986, Goldman 1979, Nagel 1977) and we have already noted, such is the nature of affirmative action and preference and the contexts within which they most frequently operate that there will be a tendency to an inverse relationship between harm and benefit.

We have, for the sake of convenience, thus far inadequately distinguished between 'wrong' and 'harm' and conducted the argument as though compensation is to be made for both or either. This may be the case but is not necessarily so. It is both possible to wrong someone without harming them and to harm them without doing them a wrong (see Fullinwider 1986: 178). In general terms we may say that to do someone a wrong is in some way to damage their interests or to violate some right that they may have (see, for example, Fried 1978: Chapter 1, Dworkin 1977a). To harm another, on the other hand, is to do them an injury, to trespass on their person or to do these things to others they hold dear (see Feinberg 1986, 1980: Chapter 3). They may also be harmed by theft or damage to things they own. A harm may be physical or psychic but ought, in general terms, to be tangible and identifiable. When we use race-conscious practices for compensatory purposes, therefore, are we compensating for wrongs done to people (or classes of people), or for the harm they have suffered (in this context, usually as a consequence of those wrongs)? The answer of course is 'for both' but we do not, in the practice of preference, distinguish between them.

Would a clearer distinction between wrongs and harm help us to answer the question about whether preference practices create 'undeserving' beneficiaries? I think it would, to the following extent. The sort of specification that the Supreme Court has recently sought – compensation for identifiable discrimination by an identifiable discriminator – presents a transparent case of making up for both wrongs done and harm suffered. Where these conditions do not apply – where arbitrarily 'selected' people benefit from preference in the absence of any immediate past acts of negative discrimination – the compensation principle has to be defended on the grounds that the moral debt of one or both of historical wrongs and ensuing harms has passed down through the generations and remains attached to present beneficiaries.

The intergenerational inheritance of moral debt does not carry equal credibility when it is attached to wrongs on the one hand and harm on the other however. As Sher has noted, the debt attaching to wrongs must at some stage be considered to have been paid[16] otherwise the history of the world becomes a history of accumulated moral debt (Sher 1981). The harm caused by past wrongs on the other hand is (or, if it is to be recompensed, ought to be) more tangible, more empirically observable. The manifest relative inequalities between racial and ethnic groups, after all, are the starting point for the entire affirmative action endeavour. It will be (and is) a matter of dispute whether the harm presently suffered by some minority groups is a linear consequence of historical (and not so historical) wrongs or of other factors, but to the extent that this is perceived as the case, then compensation would still be due. Race-conscious policies therefore are more likely to find justification in compensation for harm suffered than for wrongs done. Of course, this does not answer the question of why *these* beneficiaries and not others but it does provide another gloss on the matter. I take it that the concern about 'fortuitous beneficiaries' is either one about the moral laxity in giving benefits to the wrong people (and none to the right people) at the expense of third parties, or more simply it is about the inefficiency of race-conscious practices as instruments for compensation. The former is the more serious reservation and the second follows on from it. Are, then, the moral costs of fortuitous benefit the same whether we are talking about compensation for wrongs done or for harm suffered? The practical result will of course be the same: there will be minority gainers and losers and who they are probably will not correspond closely with who has been harmed (or wronged) and who not. But the moral price of getting the wrong (incorrect) beneficiary would seem to be less if what we are correcting for is harm suffered than if it were for a wrong done. The latter carries implications of rights or interests violated and it would be a more serious matter if those who had had rights violated (assuming for the present argument that it is not all members of a class) were not compensated (and some who had not suffered rights violation were compensated) than if the unharmed were to benefit instead of the harmed.

The purpose of this chapter has been to air some of the moral doubts and uncertainties that surround affirmative action and preference. Our aim has not been to extol a particular point of view or to argue a case for or against these practices. Many of the uncertainties to which we have given expression could be resolved with relative ease by holding to the view that all members of minority groups across the generations have suffered harm (if not wrong), and all members of the 'majority' (whites, white males) are culpable either in virtue of having been a party to the wrong-doing or of having benefited from it. The beneficiaries and cost-bearers of preference policies are then simply ciphers and their moral standing *qua* harmed and harm-doer is irrelevant. This argument seems to me to be specious and so it has been necessary to probe more deeply into the question of the distribution of guilt and injury. And although consequential reasons for preference are now more popular, the question of compensation will not, it seems, go away.

9 Equal opportunities, merits and preferences

Throughout our consideration of affirmative action and preferential treatment, we have on a number of occasions delved into the seemingly placid waters of equality of opportunity and its relation to race-conscious practices. Habitual usage lends an air of clarity and certainty to the idea; it is only when we go deeper that we find the turbulence. Because, as we have illustrated at a number of points, equality of opportunity is not an uncontestable idea, particularly when it is linked (as it must be if it is to retain any meaning-value at all) to the related concepts of the merit principle, the concept of merit, and the reward system.

The most commonly cited reason for using race-conscious practices is in order to promote more extensive equality of opportunity (as between different racial groups). And yet, as we have seen, it is the *violation* of equality of opportunity that constitutes a signal criticism of such practices when they move towards what we have called the preference end of the continuum. Our purpose here, then, is to test this last and seemingly telling argument against preference. (Lest this seems an unnecessary exercise and one that would easily be avoided by promoting only non-preference affirmative action, it should be noted once more that, given the nature of practice in America and to a lesser extent in Great Britain, this is not an available option. Preference practices are widely used and their use will in all likelihood continue to increase. We have no option but to test the morality of preference. This we have done in the previous chapter in respect of compensation; now it is the turn of equality of opportunity.)

The interaction of what we have called the 'porous concept' of equality of opportunity with the equally insubstantial notions of 'merit', the 'merit principle' and the 'reward system' makes for a bewildering complexity, and a comprehensive (and possibly still inadequate) treatment would require more than the space of one chapter. Nonetheless, we can build on the arguments already outlined, principally in Chapters 2 and 3, avoiding, so far as is possible, going over ground already covered. What will become clear, however, is that in the course of our exposition, we shall need to revise some of our earlier conclusions.

THE MORAL PRESCRIPTIVITY OF EQUALITY OF OPPORTUNITY

It appears to be axiomatic that equality of opportunity is morally apodictic. Not to afford equality of opportunities to people or groups or to violate their equality with others in pursuing opportunities is considered to be not just unfair but morally wrong, unjust, a violation of rights (see Chapter 3). From this derives the moral importance of promoting equality of opportunity through affirmative action and other measures, and equally the apparent moral wrong of violating equality of opportunity by practices of preference (and other measures). We have, however, sown the seeds of doubt about the moral force of equality of opportunity in Chapter 3. We must now nurture them a little further.

If all there was to equality of opportunity was the elimination from consideration for education or employment prospects, for example, of 'irrelevant' factors such as race, religion or sex, then there would be little ground for disputing this morally strong interpretation. It *is* morally repugnant to refuse someone a job or a place in a university *just because* they are from a minority group. But equality of opportunity, as we have seen, does not exist in isolation. It is devoid of meaning until hitched to the ideas of merit and the merit principle. Those factors or traits or abilities that we want equality of opportunity to use or exploit do not exist in a vacuum. They are valued just because they serve other purposes which may be fulfilling in themselves but are more likely to be the means to rewards – the extent and nature of which are quite beyond our sphere of influence. In other words, what constitutes 'merit', what it is that we are rewarded for possessing and exploiting, is conceptually quite independent of any process that we call equality of opportunity and yet inextricably linked to it. Furthermore, 'merit' is not a bundle of qualities of value in themselves (though we may gain satisfaction from the possession and exercise of them); they are qualities that serve other ends and their exercise is consequential. The 'best person for the job' therefore is not that person who has, and exercises, skills and talents for their own sake (and that are valued for their own sake), but rather who will apply them in a manner that will best get the job done whether it be the production of widgets or the provision of health care. Merit and its exploitation, through the merit principle, therefore, are entirely consequence-regarding and as such present us with a dilemma insofar as we might wish to support a morally strong argument for the prescriptivity of equality of opportunity (see Edwards 1990a).[1] If, therefore, as I believe is the case, equality of opportunity is devoid of meaning until linked to the substantive idea of what it is we wish to have equal opportunity to do, and if those characteristics, abilities and talents that we wish to have an equal opportunity to exploit turn out to be almost entirely consequence-regarding (in the sense of being functional for job performance), how then can we preserve the notion of the moral apodicity of equality of opportunity? The pursuit of equality of opportunity is not, it would seem, an end in itself nor indeed a moral good *per se*, but rather the means to other ends which may in *themselves* be good, but need not be and often are not (such as, for example, the maximisation of profit).

Thus far, we have posed the dilemma about the moral standing of equality of opportunity. Before we attempt to resolve it (and in the course of doing so, elucidate the consequences for preference policies), it will be necessary to make a brief detour to clarify an outstanding ambiguity.

Notwithstanding the strong consequential component to merit, value nonetheless attaches to an equality of opportunity to exercise merit characteristics both for the reward system (or the economy) and for individuals. The values are, however, quite different and of quite different kinds. So far as the economy is concerned we might assume that equality of opportunity tends to efficiency maximisation, that it is the system best designed to place the best qualified/most efficient/ most productive person in the position that most requires his or her given qualities (see for example Ansari 1987, BACIE/IPM 1987, Institute of Personnel Management 1986, Burney 1988). And, of course, this efficiency maximising potential of equality of opportunity is what underpins that favourite slogan of personnel managers, that 'equal opportunities are good for business' (Confederation of British Industry 1981, Institute of Personnel Management 1986).

Wherein, then, lies the value of equality of opportunity for the individual? The qualities that he or she possesses that are valued by the reward system, that count as meritorious (intelligence, quick-wittedness, persuasive sales patter) may be ones that he himself values, but they may not. There is no necessary compatibility between attributes valued by the reward system and attributes that we might value personally. So, we might ask, what is in it for us if all we are getting is an equal opportunity along with others to use and exploit talents that someone (or some-thing) else has attached value to? After all, I might value honesty, integrity, humility and consideration, but these are not the qualities that earn mega-salaries in the worlds of finance, banking or advertising. Now, if we ask this question at all (What is in it for me?) – and in all likelihood, most of us most of the time, do not – the answer will be an evasive one: that if we do not like the characteristics required of an effective advertising executive, we simply do not pursue a career in that direction but look for a more warm and caring role to perform, or a more creative one, or a more physical. But this does not resolve the hiatus that exists between the value that we place on certain talents and the value that the reward system places on these same talents. In a capitalist society, it is unlikely that great financial reward will attach to the exercise of talents of caring and if, therefore, we eschew the cut and thrust of advertising because we do not value the talents required for making a success of it, in favour of a more caring occupation, we shall, in all likelihood, be eschewing greater rewards too. The relative values attached to different talents and abilities, therefore, are set quite independently of any value we might attach to the talents we possess and which we want equality of opportunity to exploit. Wherein, therefore, lies the value to individuals of equality of opportunity? Why is it something to which we attach such importance?

There are a number of dimensions to an answer to this question. The first, and most general, is that we only recognise the value we place on equality of opportunity when we consider its absence. We have been here before and need not elaborate; intuitively, we feel a great harm is done when opportunities are unfairly or arbitrarily circumscribed. The reason for this is that, notwithstanding the consequential nature of the value placed on merit, equality of opportunity to exercise talents is central to our life-chances or life plans. This is reflected in differing ways in the two conceptions of equality of opportunity that we have already noted: an equality of opportunity to 'fulfil' oneself or to pursue life plans that may be definitive of the sort of person we wish to be; and second, an equality of opportunity to compete for rewards in the form of valued jobs, positions and statuses (see Chapter 3 and Edwards 1990a).

Even if, in the latter case, the competition takes place on terms other than those we might choose, we still want an equal opportunity with others to compete. So far as the former conceptualisation of equality of opportunity is concerned, we have already noted that we are here dealing with a more abstract idea and one that does not lend itself to measurement or evaluation. Our final parenthetic excursion therefore must be a brief comment on measuring equality of opportunity in respect of morally arbitrary groups.

At a case-by-case level, we may identify lack of equality of opportunity by identifying instances of discrimination which compromise it. But this quite clearly is wholly inadequate as a measure of equality of opportunity *tout court*. If we wish to know whether a particular group enjoys equality of opportunity we must necessarily have recourse to output measures that are both crude and based on a range of questionable assumptions. In short, we expect a representation of members of the groups across a range of jobs, positions and statuses that reflects their representation in the population or labour force or some other defined sub-group. The figures that we have quoted throughout earlier chapters are of this kind. As measures of equality of opportunity to *compete*, they are crude but no doubt offer some indication. As a measure of the other conception of equality of opportunity – to fulfil life plans, to pursue what to the subject is a fulfilling life – output measures are quite clearly an irrelevance unless we make the highly dubious assumption that competing for and obtaining the positions that everyone now holds is synonymous with their having fulfilled their life plans. And, of course, this applies not only to the positions that minority group members find themselves in; it applies to everyone. There just is no way of telling what the distribution across the reward system would be if everyone had had an equal opportunity to 'fulfil' themselves in terms that they value.

Does this mean then that a conception of equality of opportunity that attaches value to self-fulfilment and not to ability to compete is of little value? It certainly seems that if we attach much importance to measuring success, an equality of opportunity to fulfil plans must remain a chimera. And yet, to reject such a notion is to reject something of great value, and if equality of opportunity is to mean no more than opportunities to compete in the labour and education markets, then we have diminished its value. In fact, despite its chimerical nature, I do not believe that it makes sense entirely to reject a notion of fulfilling life plans. The fact is that for most of us equality of opportunity does not mean opportunity to compete in the abstract. Most people, in varying degrees and with differing degrees of strength, want to *do* or *be* something and they want an equality of opportunity with others, consistent with their talents and abilities to exercise that choice (see, for example, Miller 1976: Chapter 4, Braybrooke 1987: Chapters 2, 3).

There are many qualifications both conceptual and practical that must attach to the idea of life plans, career choices or conceptions of one's own good but our present requirements will be met by two general observations. The first is that some degree of symmetry will be achieved between equal opportunity to compete for positions in the reward system and equal opportunity to fulfil life plans in virtue of the fact that most conceptions of life plans or self-fulfilment will be expressed in terms of specific jobs or occupations, which are open to competition. Only rarely will people see their fulfilment to lie in doing things outwith the existing reward system (entering a closed religious order might be one example). Nonetheless, even though our life plans may be chosen from among a set of alternatives presented to us by the reward system (and though our self-fulfilment cannot usually be conceived of in independence of the reward system), the fact remains that the equality of opportunity we seek (*qua* individuals or *qua* members of a group) normally relates to an opportunity in respect of being or doing something *in particular.* If on full and mature reflection I have set my heart on being a traindriver, it is in respect of *this* that I want equality of opportunity to succeed. It is unlikely that I will be much exercised by the fact that because of my class background, my race and my sex I will suffer great *inequality* of opportunity with others of becoming an Anglican bishop.

The second point about life plans as means to self-fulfilment is the more contentious one of how much, if at all, they represent the result of free and informed choice. Would I have set my heart on being a traindriver had I been born into a different social class or gone to different schools, or been born female? (And would it matter?) Would the possibility of becoming a stockbroker or 'something else' in the City ever cross the horizon of a working-class girl from Salford? Is free choice exercised when a member of an ethnic minority group automatically rules out the possibility of a particular career or profession because of an assumption, justified or not, of the racial prejudice she will encounter? Clearly, all choices of life plan, all conceptions of what would be fulfilling for us to do, are constrained by class, family, location, sex, race, education and no doubt a host of other things. Indeed, it is impossible to conceive of an entirely free and unconstrained choice. But does it really matter? Is it not just another way of saying that we are all social beings leading lives within a social structure? Most of the time it probably does not 'matter' in the sense that there is no conceivable alternative. Where is does matter is where real possibilities to exercise talents in a fulfilling way are closed off because of arbitrary considerations of race, religion or sex.

THE RULES OF THE GAME

The apparent apodicity of equality of opportunity lies, I believe, in adherence to a set of rules for hiring, promotion and firing. Thus, in the case of hiring and promotion, it is argued that a candidate has a *right* to a position (see Chapter 8 and Goldman 1976, 1979) if he or she best fulfils a set of requirements necessary for the job to be done after due and equal consideration of all candidates.[2] There are, therefore, two components to the rules of the game: (a) due and equal consideration of all applicants; (b) a set of specified requirements to be filled.

To afford people equality of opportunity, it is necessary to treat them as equals (see Dworkin 1981). This translates in practice (sometimes slavishly), as we have seen in earlier chapters, into sets of procedures for the consideration of applications, the conduct of interviews and the comparison of relevant abilities.

Equal consideration, or treatment as equals, is a fairly abstract idea (though, morally speaking, an important one). In what respects are we to afford people equal consideration? And when we say we should treat them as equals surely this cannot mean in any and every respect? Would we wish to proceed to interview a candidate for a position in a children's home who, it transpired, had a criminal record for child abuse? What would equal consideration *mean* in such a case? Clearly, some factors are irrelevant for consideration for a post, whilst others may be highly relevant but disqualificatory. The second component of the rules of the game clearly assumes critical significance. What are 'relevant specified requirements' and what are not? These are the components of merit that we have discussed in preceding paragraphs.

The first thing to remind ourselves of is that the components of merit are consequence-regarding; they have no moral value in themselves (unlike those things that we call 'desert' such as efforts, sacrifices, hard work, diligence, conscientiousness and so on). The second thing to note is that we are too often pusillanimous in our selection of what are relevant and irrelevant factors. We admit (in the lexicon of good equal opportunity personnel practice) intelligence, quick-wittedness, track record, qualifications, confidence, self-assurance. We proscribe (again, in theory) old school tie, race, ethnicity, religion, sex, accent, connections, family, dress, brittleness, aggression (but not assertiveness). Now if 'the best person for the job' really means – as I suppose it must – 'the best person to get the job done', are we not being dishonest in prescribing only the first list and proscribing the second? Are not family connections in the police force or the army or in medicine a potential asset to someone wishing to enter these professions? Are not the connections that go with the old school tie an asset in the City? Is it not an asset to speak through your nose if you want to become a stockbroker? These are not facetious questions. The fact is that such characteristics *may* be of value given the social components of the jobs in question (and many others).

Now, if what counts as merit are those things that best get the job done (as opposed to valued characteristics of individuals *per se*) and if getting the job done is facilitated by team effort, by 'fitting in', by sharing a common sub-culture, by being a group of 'like-minded souls', as well as the characteristics on the prescribed list above, then what grounds can there be for not taking account of such things? If merit is that which is functional for job performance, then short of denying that social factors such as team spirit, common sub-culture and so on may be functional, there seems no good reason why they should not count as components of merit. This is all heresy of course. It is claiming that all those things that equal opportunities manuals say must be discounted from consideration may in fact be relevant to a consideration of how best to get a job done. But orthodoxy is Janus-faced. For what is the difference between what orthodoxy in this case abhors and what its other face promotes – namely that *diversity* is good, constructive, brings new dimensions to job performance and so on? There is no more evidence to support this (and probably less) than there is to support the efficacy of common culture and like-mindedness in getting the job done.

What, then, are the objections in equal opportunities orthodoxy to this broadening of the components of merit? The first is that it is unfair that factors such as social background and shared cultures should be taken into account, and this for two reasons. First, that such factors are irrelevant to getting the job done. I have argued that this is plain wrong – wishful thinking. Second, it is unfair because I cannot help what social class I was born into or the patterns of sub-culture with which I feel most at ease. Just because I do not talk through my nose or bray at people at drinks parties does not mean that I couldn't make a good stockbroker. This is quite true but it does not negate the fact that these things might help. But more importantly, if we are thinking of things that disadvantage me, can I any more help having been born stupid, or useless at figures, or slow-witted, or many of the other characteristics about me that personnel theory and practice *do* count as relevant to job performance? Quite simply, 'desert' *per se* will not distinguish between what orthodoxy wishes to count as relevant or non-relevant merit components. My stupidity has no more moral standing than my class background.

The second objection is more fundamental to race-conscious practice. It is that factors such as social background, 'being one of the chaps' and sharing a common sub-culture are all exclusionary and in particular they operate to exclude people of certain racial or ethnic groups. In short, they are discriminatory in effect if not in intent. But this is familiar territory and we shall trespass on it once more only very briefly. The dilemma is this. What we have called the 'rules of the game' (which, it is claimed, give certain people rights to positions) consist in two parts – a general rule of equal consideration (treating people as equals) and a set of requirements or characteristics against which we consider each applicant (the components of merit). The components of merit do not have the moral standing that we often pretend they do. They are not a set of characteristics of individuals having moral value in themselves (unlike 'desert'); they are functional requirements of job performance. This being the case, they will include factors that, in application, will have an exclusionary effect on some groups. This concerns us when the groups in question are racial, ethnic, religious or sex groups. It does not concern us when the class excluded are the chronically shy or slow-witted or the less energetic, or the awkward or the less ambitious, even though they are no more responsible for or can change their identifying characteristic than can anyone else their race, ethnicity or religious adherence. We appear, therefore, to be less than systematic in our selection of those functionally relevant characteristics we call merit, and we rule out race, religion and sex, not because they are always and automatically functionally irrelevant (though we claim this to be the case) but because intuitively we find their use in personnel decisions (and elsewhere) morally repugnant.

We may rationalise our moral disquiet at the use of race in one or both of two ways. We may wish to claim that such factors are *not* functionally relevant; they are not components of merit in the way that intelligence or quick-wittedness are. Second, we may revert to the first rule of the game and say that to allow race and religion to count is not to treat people as equals or not to afford each and every one equal consideration. The first consideration we have dealt with. The second has more substance. Now it seems to me that to allow race to count does *not* necessarily entail that people are not treated as equals. If race may count as functionally relevant or if factors that may have an adverse impact on racial groups are counted as functionally relevant, it remains possible for all applicants to be given equal consideration – to be treated as equals – in the application of the merit criteria. The fact that members of a particular group will, after due consideration, be disproportionately rejected is then simply a result of the functional requirements of the merit and reward systems. And again, it must be emphasised that what counts as merit is what is functional for job performance, *not* any inherent moral qualities of individuals.

Why then the aversion to allowing race, or any factor that may have adverse impact in these terms, to count in hiring or promotion (or other) decisions? In purely analytical terms (that is, putting aside intuition), it seems most likely that this aversion rests on a belief that, on a balance of advantages, allowing race to count has greater potential for evil than for the functional benefits that may accrue. Quite simply, it is open to too much abuse; it will allow seemingly functional arguments to cover for what are in reality decisions based on outright racial discrimination.

We have attempted, in the preceding paragraphs, to argue that the proscription on race-related factors as components of merit is logically inconsistent and stems in large measure from a reification of the idea of merit. Caution, and a little prudence, however, suggest that the intuitive aversion to letting race count is in practice a wise thing on a balance of advantage and cost. The arguments have (on purpose) been couched in terms of the potential *exclusionary* effects of allowing race to count and as such they run counter to current equal opportunities orthodoxy. But the arguments are double-edged. They may equally well be used to support a variety of race-conscious practice, including forms of preferential treatment. If we wish, for whatever reason, to reject the possibility that race-related factors may be functionally relevant to job performance, then we at the same time deny an important defence of preference – including arguments from diversity and arguments for the value of having minority group members police minority communities and for the benefit of having minority doctors or lawyers serve those communities. If, in the pursuit of equality of opportunity, we are too precious about the purity of merit, we shall find that we have rejected some valuable defences of preference practice.

Notwithstanding the inclination that we have arrived at on a balance of advantage to proscribe the use of race in hiring and promotion practices, therefore, we shall in the subsequent section examine the reverse side of the same arguments insofar as they provide support for the use of preferential treatment and affirmative action. The potential dangers of allowing race to count for the wrong reasons (such as first-order negative discrimination) must then be weighed in the balance against the anticipated benefits of preference and affirmative action.

PREFERENCE AND MERIT

It will be evident that a signal aspect of our characterisation of preference practices is their relationship to the ideas of merit and the merit principle. In practice, this will involve a consideration of the relation of preference practice to the concept of functional relevance of factors such as race to the performance of jobs.

There are two dimensions to this topic which we have not so far sufficiently distinguished. The first is that preferential treatment has in part been characterised by the use of race as if it were a component of merit itself and, therefore, a legitimate factor to take into account in hiring and promotion practices. We have come across this earlier and have called it the extension of the components of merit beyond what current orthodoxy would accept. It is this redefinition of merit that has led us to call such practice 'preferential treatment'. The second dimension covers those circumstances in which the 'preferential' hiring of minorities does not rely on arguments about the 'merit status' of race but more simply overrides the merit principle. We have called both of these strategies – incorporation into merit and the overriding of merit – 'preferential treatment'. Our main concern will be with the former if only because it requires more analysis. Overriding merit is more straightforward and we shall return to consider its 'acceptability' later in the chapter.

There are two aspects of 'incorporation in merit' that must concern us. The first is an examination of the ways and the circumstances in which race may be considered to be a component of merit alongside all the other items that we have mentioned as constitutive of the concept. This will occupy the next few paragraphs. The second aspect we shall deal with immediately and more abruptly (because an extended treatment would not illuminate our arguments further). It revolves around this assertion: that if race *were* found under some circumstances to be partly constitutive of merit, such that it could justifiably be used in job hiring and promotion, then its use under these circumstances would not constitute preferential treatment (it would have the same status as 'intelligence' or 'experience' and so on). And if this were so, it should cease to concern us except insofar that we would still need to know when and under what circumstances it *was* in part constitutive of merit (and when not). This is a perfectly reasonable line of argument but we shall not adopt it. The incorporation of race as an item of merit is, I believe, a sufficient departure from orthodox practice to require that it be afforded special scrutiny. We have adopted this view throughout in treating the expansion of merit as preferential treatment because it shifts the idea of equality of opportunity (to compete in the merit system) further from its ideal. To allow race to count introduces components of merit on which some people are not even able to compete. If being Hispanic or black is a qualification for entry to the competition then this does, I believe, constitute a sufficiently radical departure from normal practice to warrant our calling it preferential treatment. However, it must be acknowledged that the same argument will apply to other components of merit such as the old school tie or family connections. But I have no difficulty in calling these preferential treatment also.

Why should it matter then that the use of race should depend on a showing of its job-relatedness under given circumstances? Why not just override merit? There are obvious practical reasons to do with job competence and the delivery of professional services. But there are sound tactical and moral reasons too as we shall see.

The first step in our analysis must be to clarify the variety of ways in which apparently morally arbitrary characteristics such as race may be relevant to the performance of jobs or occupations in ways that would make them morally relevant criteria for selection. For present purposes we need to distinguish between three varieties of 'relevance' which we shall call 'intrinsic relevance', 'service delivery' and 'diversity'. A factor or characteristic of a person is intrinsically relevant to the performance of a job if the job could not be done or could not properly be done in its absence. Examples would include accumulated expertise, knowledge, skills and, in some instances, physical attributes like strength or the ability to work at heights. Intrinsic, functional relevance therefore is applicable to all jobs (though for some, of course, the requirements will be minimal). The second type of relevance is of less universal application but of more significance for our purposes. It might be said of jobs that contain a service element (a vast and ever increasing number and range) that in addition to, and quite separate from, the elements of intrinsic functional relevance, there will be factors, some of which influence the quality and sensitivity of the services provided. It is on these grounds, for example, that arguments are made about the need to have minority doctors or lawyers or social workers or policemen to provide services in minority communities. The extent to which the intrinsic performance element can be separately identified from this quality of provision element will vary enormously between jobs, the nature of services provided, the nature of the clientele and so on. There will often be a big overlap between intrinsic performance and service sensitivity; at other times they will be conceptually separable but in practice indistinguishable. These caveats notwithstanding, it seems clear that a real difference does exist between what is functionally relevant for a job to be done at all and what may optimise the service that the job provides. Failure to recognise this distinction has led to some dubious (if well intentioned) assertions. The arguments have never been more extensively aired than in respect of the *Bakke* decisions of 1978. Dworkin, for example, has defended the Davis affirmative action programme against claims that it violated Alan Bakke's rights and has done so on grounds that 'being black' is as morally justifiable a selection criterion as many others used by medical schools throughout the country (Dworkin 1977b). The force of his argument, however, has to rely on a confusion between what is intrinsically relevant to the practice of medicine, and what will (it is hoped) promote better health provision in black and Hispanic communities. Dworkin manages this by a sleight of hand:

> There is no combination of abilities and skills and traits that constitutes 'merit' in the abstract; if quick hands count as 'merit' in the case of a prospective surgeon, this is because quick hands will *enable him to serve the public better*, and for no other reason. If a black skin will, as a matter of regrettable fact, enable another doctor to do a different medical job better, then that black skin is by the same token 'merit' as well.
>
> (Dworkin 1977b: 14, emphasis added)

More generally, Dworkin argues that the Davis Medical School (in common with all others) was using a variety of entry requirements and assessments with the overall purpose of identifying candidates who would make useful doctors. Having a black skin was no more out of place as a selection criterion in this context than any of the others habitually used. But he is wrong in giving common identity to both manual dexterity and 'being black' as identifiers of good doctors (or even 'useful' doctors), an identity only made possible by the extraordinary weight he places on 'serving the public' as the ultimate test of value. Of course, if doctors do not ultimately 'serve the public' by healing, caring and curing, then their trade is of little value, but there are many anterior requirements for this to be done. Manual dexterity in a surgeon is one; being of a particular race or religion is not. Dworkin's argument is therefore wrong; factors such as race or religion cannot be made relevant by being brought in on the moral coat-tails of criteria, the absence of which would make the practice of medicine, if not impossible, at least a lot more rudimentary. There may well be (indeed there are) sound service-delivery related arguments for making race and religion count but they cannot be made to count as either the logical or moral equivalents of functionally necessary requirements.

It is clear that race may be a relevant factor on the part of service in affecting the quality of the service delivered, and this may constitute some form of justification for using hiring quotas – or of making membership of a particular ethnic group a requirement for the job. But what can we say about race as intrinsically relevant to job performance? We have already dismissed Dworkin's argument that there is no effective difference between intrinsic relevance and relevance to service delivery, but does this mean that race cannot be (or can only in exceptional circumstances be) of intrinsic functional relevance to job performance? The answer will in part depend, as we have noted, on the extent to which intrinsic and service-delivery relevance are separable in theory and practice. It would seem to be the case, however (and this would accord with our intuitions), that for the vast majority of jobs there is no intrinsically functional relevance in race. There are cases where there appears to be an element of intrinsic relevance but even in these there is a strong service element also. So, for example, it may well be the case that you have to be black in order to function as a social worker in a black community, not just in the sense of providing a better service to clients but more fundamentally in that the job could not be done by anyone who was not black.

Generally speaking, however, we may say that the occasions on which race is necessary for intrinsic job performance will be few and far between and, with the exception of theatrical verisimilitude, almost always linked to service provision for a particular racial group. Claims that a particular job required for its proper functioning that the operative be of a particular race would, therefore, need to be treated with some dubiety. The same is not the case in respect of service delivery. Occasions will be far more numerous when the delivery of optimal services to a minority community will require that the service deliverers be of the same ethnic group. We must next, therefore, consider whether optimal service delivery is sufficient to justify the use of race as a selection criterion; whether it becomes a functionally relevant component of 'merit' and whether, in consequence of this, its use would, or would not, constitute preferential treatment. I take it that the main point at issue would be the scope of merit. Those who see the use of race in the context of service delivery *as* preferential treatment (and a bad thing) will do so on the grounds that it stretches the scope of merit beyond what is legitimate. For those, on the other hand, who see no element of preference, this will be because whatever optimises service delivery will be a legitimate component of merit.

Does the optimisation of service delivery justify the specification of the racial group of intending job applicants? It ought not to justify such a specification for applicants to (say) medical school, as we have noted, but what about in respect of jobs for doctors in minority communities? Whether, in Dworkin's terms, 'regrettable' or not, this is, to a not inconsiderable degree, now a fact of life in the USA (and an increasingly common occurrence in Britain). In the areas of social work, medicine, law, counselling and many others, race counts in job specification and there seems to be little good reason why it should not. If it is a matter of empirical evidence that better services will be provided if the provider is of a particular racial group (or indeed that the service cannot otherwise be provided), then a specification of that group becomes a reasonable and justifiable component of the job description.

There is one final point that should be considered before we turn to look at 'diversity' as constituting job-relevance. We have argued above that if services can best be provided (and, in some instances, only be provided) by members of a particular racial group (and almost invariably because they are of the same group as the recipients) then this may justify the specification of race in job descriptions and the appointment to positions only of people of the specified group. But would being of a particular and specified racial group now constitute a part of what we call merit (as, for example, Dworkin 1977b, 1978, would seem to believe)? Can we, in other words, any longer maintain the distinction we have previously urged, between the intrinsic requirements for a job to be done, and the optimal delivery of whatever good or service it is that the job produces? However clear the distinction appears in theory, can we sustain it if the practical consequences are identical – that is, that we shall be treating race *as if* it were a component of merit? Does this not mean that the question is a rather academic one anyway? I think not. Because if we accept race as a component of merit – as relevant, that is, to job *productivity* (including performance and delivery) – then we must be prepared to accept the possibility that the embrace of merit will encompass some, or many, other factors, not all or most of which we would find as morally acceptable as race. It therefore becomes a question of whether the use of characteristics such as race for reasons of service delivery should become the basis for a broader generalisation of and incorporation into the merit principle or whether, on the other hand, each case be treated *singulatim* and incorporation for service delivery reasons not be seen as a precedent for a broadening of the 'acceptable' components of merit. The danger of allowing merit to expand to include any factor that may optimise service delivery, or for any other perceived utilitarian purpose, is that what political correctness blesses today, it may execrate tomorrow. Political correctness is undeniably in part a fashion and, as such, a poor base for moral judgements. We have only to look at the changing fortunes of Chinese Asians in the United States under first the patronage and then the perdition of the politically correct to see how fate and favours can change so quixotically (see for example Hacker 1989, Nakanishi 1989, Sowell 1990). This may be countered with the view (which we have ourselves already put) that the concept of merit is so morally inchoate anyway that it provides no intrinsic values that might enable us to decide what is, and what is not, a valid component. If old school ties are functional for job performance then why not race, religion, sex, colour, size or accent? The implications of this position for the idea of 'equality of opportunity' are far reaching but perhaps the time is due for a mild degree of apostasy over this particular icon.

Which brings us to the matter of diversity. Under the diversity argument, as we have seen in preceding chapters, it is not necessary (though it helps) to show either that a selection criterion is functionally relevant to job performance or that it optimises service delivery. Diversity is a 'value' in itself and whilst it cannot be used in complete disregard for how jobs should get done, it does not require us to agonise for too long about whether a particular criterion is intrinsic to merit or simply aids the delivery of services. That issue is circumvented by the diversity argument.

As with the other examples of job relevance, we need to ask whether diversity *per se* will justify the use of race in the allocation of jobs and positions. And we must add, does it do this independently of functional and service relevance? Two polar cases of the use of diversity will help to illustrate what is at issue. The first is the tie-break when a minority candidate is selected from among two or more equally qualified (in terms of job performance, service delivery, etc.) candidates on the grounds that for reasons of diversifying the workforce the employer has a preference for someone from an under-represented group. In the absence of the diversity question, the tie could only have been broken by the toss of a coin. The second case is less straightforward insofar as it appears to involve an employer acting in other than his or her own best interests. But since this is a matter that diversity raises in more general terms, it is worth pursuing here. In this instance we are concerned with a situation in which an employer hires minority (or other defined group) employees 'simply' because he or she wishes to promote diversity in the company, college, university, agency, etc., and does so with scant regard to other merit factors such as locating the person best qualified to perform the job, or the person best qualified on paper. This is not a description of an Alice-in-Wonderland employer: this is an employer who has elevated diversity to a much more significant position relative to other merit factors than we have habitually been used to seeing. Or, he or she may be convinced of the view that a diversified workforce is of more benefit than one chosen on the basis of what at best are merit criteria of dubious predictive performance.

We have seen already that very often rather more rhetoric than reason attaches to the promotion and use of diversity, so much so that it is sometimes hard to divine any truly unambiguous motive for its employment. Nevertheless, we can deduce from the evidence given in earlier chapters (but particularly that relating to the United States) that the promotion of diversity has little to do, ostensibly at least, with intrinsic job performance and only a little more to do with servicing communities of diverse compositions. So far as the private sector is concerned, diversity appears to have much to do with corporate image and strategy and whilst a company cannot be entirely heedless of job performance, neither in the present climate can it ignore the imperatives of diversity. Just as in earlier times large companies could not afford not to say that they were equal opportunity employers, so today must they be seen to promote diversity. The difference is that today heads are being counted. The same holds in part for universities, though as we have indicated, there is a much stronger ideological undercurrent (some might say, more like rapids) that will propel institutions down the road to diversity. This is not to assert that most or even some universities and colleges are pursuing the path of diversity either unwillingly or under duress; it is to argue, however, that neither the pace nor the extent of change has always been dictated by institutions themselves.

Does diversity constitute a component of merit? Or, to be more exact, does membership of a group that the diversity doctrine requires be more fully represented in jobs, statuses and positions constitute a part of merit? If it does not, does the hiring or promotion of minority group members in the interests of promoting diversity constitute preferential treatment in the sense that we have used this term, as appearing to override the merit principle?

Let us briefly remind ourselves of the stakes involved. If we use race as a criterion that is relevant to hiring and promoting (and laying off) staff, then we are stepping beyond those factors normally accepted as constitutive of merit (even though these may themselves be morally arbitrary). We are also, it would seem, violating the principle of equality of opportunity (to which end much of this activity is ostensibly directed). Can race-conscious practices be compatible with the promotion of equality of opportunity? And what do the arguments look like when such practices are in fulfilment of diversity?

If we are correct in our (admittedly generalised) assumption that in the private sector the pursuit of diversity has much to do with corporate image, and ultimately with competitiveness and profitability, that it is an integral part of company and corporate strategy, how then does it stand in relation to what counts as merit and an equal opportunity for all to gain, retain and advance positions? Is the use of race in these circumstances different in any fundamental way from its use in respect of optimising the delivery of services to minority communities? Both are consequence-regarding; but then so is the use of purely functional criteria such as intelligence or job skills. But the consequences are of a different kind – at least on the face of it. If the service provision arguments are valid then hiring and promoting by race (along with other factors) are means to improving the condition of minority populations. If, further, we assume that certain beneficiary minority groups are among the most deprived, then race-conscious practices in this context may be seen as justified by the needs principle (see Edwards 1987). They are, in effect, means of fulfilling one of the requirements of distributive justice. The same cannot be said when race-conscious practices are employed in the pursuit of diversity when this is part of a company or corporate strategy to promote a more 'correct' corporate image and ultimately as a means of increasing competitiveness and profitability.[3] If consequence-regarding actions, even (or especially) ones that are prima facie unjust or morally arbitrary, such as race-conscious practices, are to be judged by the nature of their ends, then clearly the promotion of diversity for corporate strategy purposes is in a different moral league to the discharge of the needs principle. We shall return to this after a brief consideration of diversity practice in universities.

We have provided something of the flavour of diversity programmes in universities in Chapter 6. The evidence presented there clearly suggests that much, and perhaps most, diversity practice in institutions of higher education is driven by ideological commitment (to equality, equality of opportunity, resource redistribution and so on), and in-creasingly, by the need to conform to the demands of a variety of types of political correctness. Again, the reasons that have been asserted for promoting racial, ethnic, sex and religious diversity in universities are many and, on occasions, fairly exotic. Thus, as we have seen, a diverse student body and faculty (and administration) are essential for the proper pursuit of scholarship; a diverse body of students and staff means a rich cultural diversity; diversity acknowledges the cultural multiplicity of American society and so on (a good example of this genre is to be found in *The Madison Plan* (University of Wisconsin-Madison 1988).) We remain sceptical about some of these claims (and in particular the one the implication of which must be that no real scholarship was possible in the USA (or Great Britain) until the 1980s when diversity was discovered), but for present purposes we shall take them at face value.

We may now ask in respect both of the private sector and of universities, do the reasons for which diversity is promoted justify the inclusion of race as a component of merit or, if not, do they justify preferential treatment as overriding merit? So far as the private sector is concerned, this may be stated more crisply in the following terms; does the pursuit of corporate strategy justify the use of race as an item of merit? (Is 'merit' whatever conduces to corporate strategy?) If corporate strategy *per se* does not permit us to extend the bounds of merit beyond what conventional usage permits, does it allow us to override the merit principle?

There is a temptation to answer the former question in the affirm-ative. Once we have acknowledged that merit is those things that 'get the job done best' (and what is conducive to getting the job done best *may* count as merit),[4] then all that remains to be done is to make 'corporate strategy' and 'getting the job done' synonymous or at least consistent ends. Thus, if what counts as merit includes characteristics that are functionally relevant to job performance and which optimise the delivery of services, it is but a short step to argue that merit is also whatever promotes company and corporate strategies provided these are legal and pursued by legal means. If this reasoning is sustainable, then hiring by race in pursuit of diversity is consistent with the merit principle. And if the corporate strategy requires a hiring or promotion quota for one or more racial groups then this is permissible within the bounds of the merit principle.

These are arguments that it is difficult to counter (short, that is, of denying the premise) but the consequences will remain unpalatable to many – and illegal in process in both countries we have examined. So, let us move on to the next step which requires, for the sake of argument, that diversity does *not* permit the incorporation of race as components of merit. That being so, does the pursuit of diversity in fulfilment of part of a corporate strategy permit the violation of the merit principle (and of the idea of equality of opportunity) by requiring the preferential hiring and promotion of minority group members? Legally speaking of course the answer is 'no'; diversity is no defence against legal or constitutional charges of discrimination. In practice, as we have seen, and particularly in the United States, the legal proscription has not been sufficient to prevent the use of considerations of race in recruitment and promotion. Indeed, if diversity is to be pursued aggressively, and if the incorporation of race as a component of merit is denied, then policies of preference for minority group members which override merit must be an inevitable means to this end.

The focus of this chapter has been on the idea of equality of opportunity and its relation to race-conscious practices. Along the way it has been necessary to direct attention to the related concepts of merit and the merit principle. It is now time to pull together some of these threads. Equality of opportunity, it has been argued, can only properly be understood in relation to the separate but connected ideas of the merit principle and the components of merit itself. Divested of these, it is devoid of meaning. We cannot therefore consider the relation of race-conscious practices to equality of opportunity without also con-sidering the natures of merit and the merit principle.

Race-conscious practices (or what we have called the preferential treatment end of the continuum, the other end of which is mild affirmative action) have been characterised in two ways for present purposes (there are others). First, such practices may incorporate into the body of components that make up merit, characteristics (notably race) that normally would be excluded. Quite simply, therefore, race-conscious practices will allow race to count in procedures of hiring, promotion and firing. Standard personnel practice, and the law, forbid this in both countries we have examined. Second, race-conscious practices may make no pretence at incorporating novel components into merit and may simply override the merit principle by allowing race to count quite independently of any more orthodox personnel procedures.

Our characterisation of merit, here and elsewhere (see Edwards 1990a, 1990b), has been of a set of characteristics attaching to people which are relevant in some way to how a job or a task is performed. The components of merit have no moral value in themselves (as would be the case with the components of desert); they have value for purely consequential reasons – namely, the contribution they can make to getting jobs and tasks done. It is in consequence of this that it has been necessary to specify more clearly the ways in which the components of merit are functionally relevant to job performance. In particular, it has been necessary to show how race might be relevant to job performance *if* it was to be counted a component of merit. Three broad categories of relevance were identified (as much for their currency of usage as for any theoretical reason): intrinsic functional relevance, reasons of optimal service delivery and diversity.

This has been the groundwork of the chapter. The rest has been concerned with whether equality of opportunity is compromised or, on the other hand, promoted by preference practice in either its 'incorporation into merit' or its 'overriding of merit' forms. The answers to these questions, we have maintained, will differ in respect of the three types of relevance.

Insofar as preferential treatment as the incorporation of race into merit is concerned, there seems little danger of serious violence to equality of opportunity being done, given the morally inchoate nature of the characteristics that are habitually counted as merit. Race may in some circumstances be just as relevant to job performance as family connections, networks, sub-cultures and so on. This will apply far less, however, to intrinsic functional relevance than to either service delivery or diversity. The danger, of which we must always be aware, is that letting race count can cut both ways, and hence our reticence as noted earlier.

Where race-conscious policies take the form of overriding merit (with no pretence to functional relevance), the picture is less clear (or even more murky). It would seem that, in respect of intrinsic functional relevance, equality of opportunity cannot be served by appointing by race in complete disregard for the abilities, talents and qualifications deemed necessary, or at least desirable, for the proper performance of the job. There are many components to *inequality* of opportunity and race is one of them. The same must in general be true for relevance to service delivery, where equality of opportunity would presumably mean appointing that candidate best able to deliver optimal services to the community in question. An overriding of other relevant factors in favour only of race could not but violate the idea of equality of opportunity (as well as compromising service delivery).

In the case of diversity, however, it has to be said that insofar as it is treated as a value in itself (and an end worth pursuing in its own right) then the overriding of traditional merit criteria is neither here nor there, and equality of opportunity becomes a matter of statistical representation rather than individual rights to positions. And, it has to be said, in many occupations it would not matter in terms of job performance which of these two variants of equality of opportunity was used.

But what of rights? We raised, but did not resolve, the question of rights in Chapter 8. The tentative conclusions we have reached above now force us to re-examine the force of rights-arguments in relation to equality of opportunity. What makes the conclusions we have drawn here tentative is that they must face the immediate rejoinder that to allow race either to count as a component of merit, or to override merit through preference practices, necessarily violates the rights of those who would have got a job or position, or received promotion, on the basis of being the best person for the position according to the established and accepted canons of the merit principle. It is this assumption of rights-violation that gives force to the 'innocent victims' argument. Furthermore, there seems to be a good deal of intuitive strength to Goldman's argument that without there being rights-to-positions in virtue of being the best qualified, there remains little with which to counter first-order negative discrimination and that the idea of equality of opportunity begins to look hollow (Goldman 1979). Both arguments, but in particular the latter, are less forceful than they at first appear.

What then is the basis for the claimed rights-to-positions of the most competent? It would seem to lie in the following factors: that those things that make up 'merit' – and the merit principle itself – are largely correct, justifiable and agreed upon by all who have an interest; that task performance (in the sense of getting the job done) is widely valued as an end to pursue; that there is general agreement on what constitutes competence and job-doing; that the best person in some sense 'deserves' the position (because they have worked or studied hard, or made sacrifices); and that if everyone has equality of opportunity then the merit system will position everyone in their 'rightful' place in the reward system. All these assumptions are unsound. We have said enough about merit and the merit principle to throw doubts on the first point. It is possible that there is a general agreement that task performance is useful but it is by no means universal. Ideas about competence and job-doing certainly would not command general agreement in a multi-cultural society. It cannot in general be said that we deserve positions; certainly desert *is* a component, but much of what makes up merit is not, as we have seen, constitutive of desert. Finally, we would all occupy our 'rightful' place in the reward system if there were pure equality of opportunity and merit consisted only of those things that we could be said to deserve. (Otherwise, our 'rightful place' would in part be determined by genetic factors which most of us would probably not think to be constitutive of rights.)

The grounding of rights in merit and the merit principle, therefore, appears less than compelling. But there remains Goldman's second point that there is little to equality of opportunity if the person it throws up as the best qualified in the competition does not have a right to the prize. The difficulty with this argument is that it makes the value of equality of opportunity contingent upon rights to positions but says nothing about how compelling these rights must be for equality of opportunity to be fully valuable and valued. Clearly, if positions and jobs and statuses were allocated alphabetically by family name, there would be little room for a concept of equal opportunities. We are talking of arrangements in which the idea of equality of opportunity is (at least ideally) possible. But if its value is to inhere in something called 'rights to positions', however jejune that turns out to be, then equality of opportunity itself becomes contaminated by the same moral arbitrariness. We cannot tie equality of opportunity so closely to an imperfect merit system. What matters is that we have less than equality of opportunity, *and* a merit system that is in some measure arbitrary in its moral effects. They are closely connected but there is no reason why progress in one must be contingent upon the other.

If the merit system does not bestow on us rights-to-positions, what *can* we expect from it? Or can we 'expect' nothing from the process of applying for and competing with others for a job or position? The rules of the merit game are not entirely quixotic; they do set up certain expectations but that is probably as far as they do go. They do not give us a right nor even an entitlement to positions, but rather a 'reasonable expectation' of being awarded a position under certain sets of circumstances. Expectations of course may more easily be overridden than rights.

10 Tailored preference

Should preference be given to people from minority ethnic or racial groups when job vacancies are being filled, promotions made, lay-offs imposed and places in universities allocated? The groundswell of opinion that would answer this question affirmatively is moved by the conviction that such minorities are victims – of history, of circumstance and (mainly) of the majority population. It is a conviction that fuels much equal opportunities and race relations work and which underpins a substantial amount of research on matters concerning race. Particularly is this the case in Great Britain. This makes for an ideologically charged environment both for practice and for research in which disinterested (not uninterested) work can all too readily be labelled as reactionary, racist or 'religionist' or sexist, or any combination of these. Perhaps it is wrong, in an area where great injustices have occurred, to be anything other than committed to a reformist view, but this is not conducive to improved knowledge and better understanding, which in the longer term must be more contributive to greater justice than will ideological rhetoric.

In the foregoing chapters, we have mustered some data and a good many arguments about affirmative action and preferential treatment. Some of these have been arguments in favour of such practices; others have been critical. In sum, they provide no firm conclusion to our opening question. Such apparent agnosticism falls short of that commitment which (in the rhetoric of race) divides those who are a part of the solution from those who are part of the problem. It is probably worse than a full-blown derogation of preference practices. It is time, therefore, to take stock of the morality of preference.

In what has gone before, we have tried not to (or not tried to) make out a systematic case for or against affirmative action and preference. Nor shall we do so here. Rather, our purpose is to summarise and weigh up the main arguments for and against, and from this process derive a view about whether morality and practical results argue for race-conscious practices.

Prefatorily, it needs to be said that arguments will not be consistent across the entire continuum from affirmative action to preferential treatment. Practices nearer to the affirmative action end will in general be more widely acceptable though even they will not be costless as some would maintain. Arguments about preferential treatment will need to be stronger and sounder because such practices appear to do more violence to justice and attract more opprobrium in consequence. We may assume, therefore, that an adequate defence of a preference policy will *ipso facto* make its weaker affirmative action version also defensible.

THE PURPOSES OF PREFERENCE

Whether we can find affirmative action or preference practices to be justified and hence, in the face of counter-arguments, permissible will depend in large measure on the purposes for which they are used. If there are circumstances in which the demands of justice can best be met or only be met by using race-conscious practices, then there must be compelling reasons for not doing so. Such compelling reasons would include the creation of even greater injustices by the use of such practices. The two main apodictic grounds for the use of preference, as we have seen, are compensating for the harm and violated rights caused by past discrimination and oppression, and the ensuring of equal opportunities where these are compromised. Violation of rights gives rise to a right to compensation and inequality of opportunity to a right to have needs met (including the removal of discriminatory barriers).

There are a variety of consequential reasons why we might want to pursue preference policies, but in general, practices that are prima facie unjust will not so easily be justified on the grounds of consequence as by the demands of justice itself. Three types of consequential reason have been identified: those consequences that are intended to benefit the minority group in question; those the benefits from which lie elsewhere (foreign investment, civil peace, company image and so on); and third, 'diversity', which, because of its iconic status, particularly in the United States, is worthy of mention in its own right. Of course, diversity itself is pursued for a variety of reasons, some of which are intended to benefit the affected minorities while others have more to do with marketing strategies, company image, the constraints of labour demographics and the pressure of political correctness. Other things being equal, I take it that we would find preference practices more easily justified by some of these purposes than others.

AGAINST PREFERENCE

It will be necessary only to rehearse the main arguments against the use of preference (and, to a lesser extent, affirmative action). They are the following. First, insofar as preference is used as a means of compensating for past harm, it is wrong because it must assume whole-group harm and whole-group guilt. It requires that all whites (or white males) are guilty (in virtue of receiving benefit if not from causation) and that all minority group members have been wronged and harmed. These assertions are not true. Furthermore, such injustice is compounded by the quixotic way in which preference practices select those who benefit and those who bear the costs. Affirmative action and preference practice are, therefore, singularly inefficient ways of righting past wrongs. Indeed, they create more injustice than they could ever correct.

We have seen that the argument from compensation has been less in evidence over the past ten years in America (it was never a strong argument in Great Britain) and has been replaced in large measure by 'diversity'. The prime reason for this, I believe, is that a defence of preference on the grounds of compensation for past harm has become less and less compelling. The counter-arguments outlined above have commanded more support than proponents of preference have been able to cope with. Notwithstanding this, the Supreme Court in America has seen fit still to treat preference practice as a matter of compensation and not of equality of opportunity or diversity. And in the issue of compensation, it found an easy target. Unlike the Court, however, it is possible to believe that while preference is a poor tool for effecting compensation, that does not mean that some compensation is not due. But to argue that race-conscious policies can effect compensation in any distributively just way as between the members of minority groups and between them and majority groups is simply neither compelling nor convincing. We shall come across another reason for thinking this in subsequent paragraphs. Whilst it has to be said, therefore, that some compensation remains due to some groups in some circumstances, there is strong evidence that preference and affirmative action are not an appropriate means of effecting it.

The second argument against preference concerns the moral (and personal) costs involved in its overriding the merit principle and violating people's rights to positions. This argument must be considered in respect both of the promotion of equality of opportunity and of consequential reasons for pursuing preference. (If the moral costs cannot be justified in respect of the morally apodictic grounds of promoting equality of opportunity, even less are they likely to be justified on grounds of consequence, and even less if the consequence is not a direct benefit to the affected group.) We need not elaborate on this argument further. In a nutshell, it is that merit and merit alone should count in hiring and promotions. To take anything else into consideration is unjust. It also overrides rights to positions, is dangerous, corrosive and politically suicidal.

There are many other more tangential arguments against preference that enter on the coat-tails of these two critiques, but we need not re-rehearse them here. Two other concerns must, however, be considered which arise not from a moral critique of affirmative action and preference, but from the way in which they have been applied. It will be clear from the examples we have described in earlier chapters of affirmative action and preference in Great Britain and the United States that, whilst there are some variants, the body of practice is broadly similar in both countries, for all groups and all purposes.[1] We have called affirmative action and preferential treatment variously 'policies' and 'practices'. In application, however, they begin to look more like a bag of tools to be brought out as and when occasion or ideology demand. This gives rise to two difficulties: that the same bag of tools is brought out and used indiscriminately whatever and however many the groups involved and whatever are the purposes being pursued.

In areas where there is only one or largely one minority group, the indifference of affirmative action to different groups will hardly matter. Where, on the other hand, a number of different groups will be affected (West Indian, Indian, Pakistani, or – in the United States – African-Americans, Hispanics, Chinese Asians and so on) it will matter a great deal. We cannot assume, for example, that the same affirmative action and preferential treatment practices – of the kind we have identified in both public and private sector agencies – will have an identical impact on all minority ethnic groups. This is an as yet unresearched area but it seems reasonable to speculate (and there is some evidence already cited of differential impact) that affirmative action and preferential treatment practices will *not* have the same effects on each group. To assume a common impact from outreach, targeted advertising, race-norming selection procedures, targeted training and so on is to assume common histories for all groups, identity of first languages, extent of disadvantage and past and present discrimination, a unity of cultures and identical demographic structures. None of these assumptions is tenable. Some racial and ethnic groups will benefit more than others from identical preference practices and if those that benefit less are already more deprived than other groups, such practice will serve to increase inequalities between different minority groups and between some of them and the majority. In short, inter-group equality will not be served by affirmative action and preference practices that remain untailored.

Closely related to the above arguments and constituting our fourth case against race-conscious practices is the fact that as well as being indifferent to different groups, such practices are also indifferent to the purposes for which they are being pursued. Just the same instruments are applied whether the purposes are compensation for past harm, the promotion of equality of opportunity, the pursuit of diversity or any number of other more consequential ends. This cannot be a realistic strategy. And the inequities it produces are compounded by the widespread habit of allowing substitutability between groups in monitoring the achievements of goals or quotas, as if all minority groups count the same in terms of inequality of opportunity and degree of compensation due. We have noted, for example, that some of the agencies we have studied in Great Britain and the United States, whilst monitoring their workforce composition in terms of each constituent minority group, would aggregate all groups into an 'ethnic minority' category for the sake of counting minority gains. The bizarre situation may arise, therefore, where compensation for past harm to African-Americans may be paid by hiring more Hispanic workers simply because that is the serendipitous result of applying affirmative action and preference practices. Clearly the types of practice that will be most appropriate to effect compensation for harm will need to be very different to those the purpose of which is to promote equality of opportunity. Current policy and practice in Britain and America are largely blind to this distinction.

The first two of these cases against affirmative action and preference are arguable. The second two must stand as serious weaknesses in current practice. If there is a case for preference (or practices at the preference end of the continuum), there must be an equally strong case for its reform so that practice will discriminate between groups and between purposes.

FOR PREFERENCE

The first argument in favour of preference is a defence against its principal critique – that it is unjust because it necessarily involves overriding the merit principle and violating people's rights to positions by competence. We have argued this matter at some length and have found that in some circumstances the criticism is not sustainable. The merit principle is entirely ends-regarding; there can be nothing morally prescriptive about it. What counts as merit we have found to be largely morally arbitrary, such that no damage would be done to justice or rights if race was counted as an item of merit where there was good reason for doing so. There is no substance in the argument, therefore, that great moral harm would be done if race was sometimes an item of merit or if at times the merit principle was overridden by racial preference. This is particularly the case when we are pursuing equality of opportunity but it will not help us to counter the critique in relation to compensation. That remains strong.

Incorporating race or religion in merit or overriding the merit principle are more dubiously justified when the purpose is consequential rather than deontic. In general we have argued that if the purpose is to benefit minorities or minority communities, this would constitute sufficient grounds for overriding merit. If, on the other hand, the purpose does not involve intentional benefit for minorities (even though they may in practice benefit) but rather such things as company image, maintaining foreign investment, keeping civil order, the slavish pursuit of political correctness or massaging a political image, then it seems that the moral costs (there must be *some* in overriding merit) will be too high for preference to be justified. Both beneficiaries and victims will be merely instruments for some other purpose.

The second main argument for preference is that it is quite simply in the face of the failure of orthodox policy the *only* way to compensate for harm, create more equality of opportunity, more racial equity and equality. If we do not sanction affirmative action and preference, so this argument goes, all these injustices will remain. It was indeed, as we have seen for both countries that we have examined, the failure of 'colour-blind' policies to effect any significant improvement in the condition of minorities that led to the introduction of policies that did take minorities into account.

The argument rests upon an assumption that inequalities (and inequities) remain after thirty years of affirmative action in the United States and fifteen or so years in Great Britain. If this is true (and it is), it must be an indictment not only of orthodox practice but of the effectiveness of affirmative action and preference as well. The response to this could well be that we have only toyed with race-conscious practice and that if it is to have substantial impact, it must be pursued with far more vigour. But this is too gloomy a diagnosis. Inequalities do remain, but significant progress has also been made – at least in the United States, where the quality of data enables us to measure change.[2] Thus, for example, in the private sector of the economy in America the employment participation rate[3] for all minorities combined increased from 11.2 per cent in 1966 to 21.4 per cent in 1988. For blacks it rose from 8.2 per cent to 12.4 per cent, for Hispanics from 2.5 per cent to 6.2 per cent, and for Asians and Pacific Islanders from 0.3 per cent to 2.4 per cent – an eight-fold increase.[4] There were similar – though slightly lower – increases in the public sector.[5] The Equal Employment Opportunity Commission attributes much of this increase to the effect of affirmative action practice (as a government agency, it cannot acknowledge any effects due to preferential treatment) (Equal Employment Opportunity Commission 1989b). The examples of American practice that we have provided lend some support to this view – though preferential treatment emerges there as an important driving force.

Race-conscious practices of the sort we have described are not the only ones that will have an impact on the condition of minority groups. There are other programmes in the fields of education, housing, income support and pre-school provision which are at least partially targeted at minorities. But affirmative action and preferential treatment do constitute the most significant and effective race-conscious policies particularly in the field of employment. There is evidence that these practices do work (even if imperfectly). Without them, minority representation in all levels of employment would be considerably less than it is. This must constitute, therefore, a strong argument in their favour.

The third argument in favour of preference is a simple one. It is that the costs of preference are worth bearing if the consequences are good. If, therefore, preference policy does compensate for past harm, does reduce inequalities of opportunity, does conduce to racial equality and equity and does improve the quality of life of minority group members, then the costs in terms of injustice performed, violated rights, the creation of innocent victims and so on are worth bearing. But this is no more than an assertion of which way the balance will tilt when we weigh the costs and benefits. It is asserting the answer before doing the sums.

THE LIMITS OF PREFERENCE

Any evaluation of the benefits and costs of preference must take account of the limits to its effectiveness. There are two dimensions to these limits – the boundaries beyond which it is inoperative, and the limits to effectiveness imposed by the nature and aetiology of the problems it is designed to tackle. The first is more easily dealt with than the second.

Affirmative action and preference practices operate primarily in employment, higher education and (to a lesser extent) in business set-asides. Of and by itself, it cannot touch many other components of the relative deprivation of minority groups such as poor and overcrowded housing, poor (or no) education, chronic poverty and insecurity, inadequate health care, and for some members of some minority groups, an environment of crime and drug-dealing and drug-taking. Getting a job (through a preference programme) will certainly help to alleviate some of these, but the causal connection is a distant one. We should be careful how much we claim for race-conscious policies.

At the very beginning, we noted that the point of departure for affirmative action was the evident inequalities between racial and religious minorities and majority populations. In the field of employment this was evidenced by higher levels of unemployment and by under-representation in professional and managerial positions. We have also noted the tendency, in Britain in particular, to attribute these inequalities in large measure (and for some, entirely), to racial discrimination. It is this, more than anything else, I believe, that has led us to expect more of affirmative action and preference than they are capable of delivering. These practices are best at removing discriminatory barriers and compensating[6] for the effects of past discrimination (by, for example, training programmes). If it is true, therefore, that employment inequalities are largely or entirely due to discrimination, then affirmative action and preference practice ought to be highly effective. But it isn't and they are not (though they are effective in some measure as we have seen). Employment inequalities are the result of a multiplicity of factors of which discrimination is but one. Differences in cultural predilections, age structures, career choices, social class, mobility and location will all have an effect on employment patterns along with discrimination. And affirmative action can do little if anything to correct for these effects.

CAN PREFERENCE BE JUSTIFIED?

In many circumstances it can.[7] Practices that fall at the affirmative action end of the range, even though they are not costless, will command wide acceptance. It is those that practise preference that are less than (officially) popular. However, I doubt that any significant difference between the two can be sustained for long.

If we wish to support preference practices we must surmount two hurdles. The first is that they override the merit principle and violate rights to positions by competence. The second is that as an instrument for compensation they are singularly inefficient given the arbitrary way in which it distributes burdens and benefits. We have argued that the merit principle and the concept of merit itself carry no moral prescriptivity and that any 'rights' they bestow are illusory and should more correctly be called 'legitimate expectations' (but which should, nonetheless, be overridden only for assured good cause). Provided that the ends are just (or at least not venal), therefore, there is no morally strong argument against including race as a component of merit. There is a caveat however. As to the question of the unsuitability of preference as a compensatory instrument, this remains a telling criticism. It probably creates more intra-group injustices than any compensatory effects it might have can justifiably support. However, I do not think that the argument for or against preference can any longer be decided on the issue of compensation. It just is not a compensatory mechanism and we should drop any pretence that it is.

The caveat to our qualified support of preference practice is that we take note of the other two counter-arguments. Supportable practice must be more sensitive and tailored to differences between groups and to the purposes for which is it being used. Different levels of under-representation between different groups, for example, must be reflected in the way that preference practice is implemented.

Finally, we must be careful of the reasons for using preference before we incur its inevitable costs. Promoting equality of opportunity, improving services to minorities, improving their quality of life and promoting equity between groups will justify the imposition of more costs (on 'innocent victims') than will consequences that have little or nothing to do with beneficiary minorities and more to do with company image, political correctness or party political advantage.

DIVERSITY AND EQUALITY OF OUTCOME

What do we hope to achieve by the use of affirmative action and preferential treatment? The short-term aims are clear enough; they are to increase minority group representation across the reward system. (Other race-conscious policies, it is hoped, will pursue related ends but we confine our remarks here to what has been at the focus of this work.) There is a danger, however, that statistical representation will (indeed already has) become totemic – an ultimate end, with longer-term goals lost sight of. This matters because there is reason to think that equivalent representation of all groups across the reward system is not in itself an adequate or proper end for preference practices. It has the merit of being measurable but that may be a danger in itself if what is measured is a statistical artefact.

Equivalent statistical representation appears to be what those who argue for equality of outcome wish to see. (If it isn't, then it is not clear what exactly they are arguing for. There are a multitude of dimensions to group equality – in respect of status or income, wealth, consideration, dignity, citizenship and so on, but with the exception of income none of these is necessarily coterminous with equivalent representation across the reward system.) The difficulty is not that equivalent representation is necessarily a bad or unworthy end to pursue, but rather that it might be an artificial end, chosen because it is measurable but unrealisable because of its artificiality.

Would we, in a world from which discrimination and its effects had been banished, expect to find equivalent statistical representation of all racial groups (and all other morally arbitrary groups) across the entire reward system? We have already noted in Chapter 3 a multiplicity of reasons that help to sustain inequality of opportunity, and discrimination in its various forms is but one of these. But even given equality of opportunity, is it not possible – to put it no higher – that this multiplicity of factors would also produce inequality of outcome – or, in the absence of any wrong-doing, *difference* in outcome? For it would be wrong in the absence of wrong-doing and harm to equate unjustified inequalities with legitimate differences. Furthermore, we do acknowledge that differences are a worthwhile thing to work for – at least I take it that that is what the diversity movement is all about. Why then do we 'celebrate diversity' and at the same time expect sameness of outcome and particularly as this is measured by equivalent statistical representation? Are we consistent in celebrating a diversity of cultures, traditions, races, religions, art forms and histories among the population while at the same time expecting all members of all traditions to make the same career, job and life-plan choices? Because if they do *not* then we cannot possibly expect equivalent statistical representation. So, if choices were made by all members of all groups under the same degree of constraints (we must assume that completely unconstrained choices are not possible in the labour and education markets) in a world of diversity, can we expect all groups to make similar choices or is it realistic to think that there will, in all likelihood, be some systematic group differences? The latter proposition seems at least as plausible as one that argues for identity of choice.

There is a very real possibility, therefore, that celebrating diversity and promoting statistical parity are incompatible. The pursuit of statistical parity may be a worthwhile interim goal, indicative of one kind of equality, but it is a limited goal. There are many dimensions to equality and many of these recognise difference as a component of equal freedoms. If we can acknowledge that difference and a wider conception of equality are compatible, and mutually reinforcing, aims, then we may begin to see preference practice in a more accommodating light.

Meanwhile, the more distant view remains blurred. If, in Britain, for example, we were to implement preference policies, we would continue to measure their success in terms of the distribution of minorities across the occupational system and of differential unemployment rates. But we would not know when to stop because we have no vision of how things *should* look. Perhaps an equality of dignity and respect between all racial and ethnic groups is as near as we can get to a picture of what a racially just society should be like. If that is so, then we shall have to put time limits on our use of preference. We cannot hope to engender respect and dignity by the long-term use of practices which are based on an assumption (albeit a true one) that minority groups are always and ever the victims of discrimination and oppression. Casting minorities always as victims may work for a while, but it will not, in the long term, engender respect. Indeed, oppression-talk will turn out to have been more functional for white liberals in need of a cause than for equality of opportunity and respect for all.

Appendix: A note on methodology

The approach used in Chapters 4 and 6 is not that of case studies in its usual sense. The purpose of the material gathered from a number of institutions in Great Britain and the United States of America is to illustrate arguments developed elsewhere in the book and to provide examples of the development, organisation and practice of affirmative action. It has not been the intention to provide detailed and comprehensive analyses of each institution. The quantity and quality (and usefulness) of the numerical data made available by the institutions examined was very variable and has again been used for illustrative purposes. In some cases it was possible to estimate changes in minority representation in workforces over time but in others – even where sophisticated affirmative action programmes were in place – the data required to do this were not available.

THE SELECTION OF ORGANISATIONS

Selection criteria were few in number and were determined in large measure by the need to identify a range of affirmative action practice. It was not the intention to examine organisations that did little by way of promoting equality of opportunity – even though this could have been of value in itself. The first objective, therefore, was to find organisations that were active in promoting equality of opportunity and in using affirmative action. In both Great Britain and the United States it was evident that both public and private sector organisations were actively pursuing equal opportunities by means of affirmative action policies and, given their different functional aims and responsibilities, these may well have been distinctive in style and content and so, in order to capture any such differences, organisations from both sectors were included.

Organisations in Great Britain for inclusion in the study were selected on the basis of reputation. A shortlist was drawn up of organisations that received frequent mention in the equal opportunities, race and personnel literature as being ones that were active in the pursuit of equal opportunities and the use of affirmative action. Initial approaches were made to ten local authorities and eight large private institutions in anticipation of 'enrolling' five from each sector. There were some outright rejections and two companies declined to co-operate after discussions were held with them. The majority of the refusals were on the grounds of the time commitment required or (in three cases) that they were already co-operating (or had recently co-operated) in research. It is worth noting, however, that two local authorities refused co-operation on the grounds that the research was being conducted by a white male. In the event, agreement was reached with six local authorities and four private sector organisations in Great Britain.

Selection of organisations in North America was facilitated by colleagues at the College of Urban Affairs and Public Policy at the University of Delaware but the number that could be covered was determined by time constraints. Detailed information was collected in one large company, at two levels of government (state and city) and in one university, and supplementary information was gathered in two further universities and at federal government level.

The terms and conditions of co-operation were agreed with each organisation before work began and for a small number the maintenance of anonymity was a prior condition of co-operation. Rather than adopt the somewhat unsatisfactory expedient of identifying some respondent organisations whilst maintaining the anonymity of others, therefore, all have been identified solely by alphabetic cipher. Likewise individual respondents remain anonymous.

THE DATA

An average of four meetings was held in each organisation in Great Britain, and three per organisation in the United States. In all instances, discussions were held with the person responsible for equal opportunities, affirmative action or personnel matters, and where other personnel had an interest in or knowledge relevant to an understanding of affirmative action practice in the organisation, these also were interviewed. All the discussions were guided by a check-list of required information and transcripts prepared of the substance of each discussion. Wherever possible, however, documentary support was requested on topics such as the equal opportunity policy, organisational structure, the line-management of the policy, departmental responsibilities and so on. Copies of all relevant data on minority group representation, changes over time, and the results of any monitoring exercises were also requested, and, in almost all instances where they were available, were obtained.

The transcripts of interviews were used alongside documentary evidence, to provide an account of affirmative action and equal opportunities, but for narrative reasons direct quotations from transcripts are kept to a minimum. Documentary material has been used more extensively for quotation purposes.

Only rarely have data provided by respondent organisations been reproduced in their original and complete form. Rather, they have been used as the material from which to derive the most germane and illustrative information. As much as possible of the useful data has been incorporated in the tables.

Notes

1 WHEN RACE COUNTS

1 Of course, affirmative action and preferential treatment may be used in respect of any morally arbitrarily defined groups such as women or homosexuals. Our interest here is solely with race.

2 This is not to say that policies ought not to be sensitive to the different needs of separate groups.

3 Relatively deprived groups are not always minority groups – they can constitute a majority of the population (see Sowell 1990).

4 This is a broad generalisation which in some particulars would be untrue. Indian Asian groups in Great Britain and Chinese Asian groups in the United States have made social and economic progress, both absolutely and relatively, compared with the majority group and with other minorities (see Brown 1984, Steele 1990b, Smith and Welch 1986, Hacker 1989). As a general statement about the relative positions of different minority groups and the majority, it remains true, however.

2 THE NATURE AND VARIETIES OF AFFIRMATIVE ACTION

1 Race-conscious policy is our present concern but other groups – and in particular gender and religious groups – are also the subject of affirmative action practice. Much of what follows on the theory of affirmative action will apply equally to other affected groups.

2 'Racial disadvantage' is not a technical term. As in so much of the language of race relations, the term is more declamatory than informative. One interpretation would be that members of ethnic minorities suffer to a greater extent than the majority population from a range of social and economic deprivations including housing, education, environment, health, employment and unemployment, and poverty. This in turn might mean that a greater proportion of minority group members than of the majority group suffer such deprivations, *or* that they suffer from them to a greater extent, or both. Second, it may mean that minority group members suffer from a different and distinct range of deprivations that give rise to *special* needs. Third, it may mean that either of these two conditions is compounded by racial discrimination. Most authoritative studies (House of Commons 1981, Brown 1984, Smith 1977) collapse all three interpretations into one. For many purposes this might not matter. It does matter if the purpose is to devise effective counter-measures. In what follows the term is used more selectively.

3 Patterns of representation differ of course as between different ethnic minority groups.

4 There are many more. The four mentioned here are salient to a derivation of affirmative action. Others will be considered in subsequent chapters.

5 Elaboration of differences between group and individual equality of opportunity is to be found in Loury (1987), Simon (1977) and Sher (1987).

6 Though discriminated against groups are defined with varying degrees of precision.

7 Besides those already mentioned, derivations of material principles of distributive justice have been made by Benn and Peters (1959), Frankena (1962), Honoré (1968), Lucas (1980), Perelman (1963), Rescher (1966), Ross (1974), Vlastos (1962), Von Leyden (1963), Braybrooke (1987).

8 It is worth noting the absence of handicap from this list. Although the subject of equal opportunities and sometimes of affirmative action, handicap is not a morally arbitrary criterion insofar as it will almost always imply greater or different needs *by definition*. Action in respect of the handicapped therefore is fully in accord with the needs principle. For further discussion of morally relevant and arbitrary criteria in the context of affirmative action, see Nickel (1977), Goldman (1975), Cowan (1972), Bayles (1973a), Taylor (1973).

9 The compensatory argument for affirmative action in the US has less currency today however than it did ten to fifteen years ago (see Belton 1981, Mishkin 1983). It is not an argument that has ever gained much popularity in Great Britain either.

10 Although the same practices are referred to when 'preferential treatment' and 'reverse discrimination' are used in the US, the latter term is more often applied in a denunciating fashion and is meant to convey the meaning 'discrimination *against* whites or males'.

11 At this stage, the discussion is hypothetical. The use of quotas is illegal in Great Britain, and in America may only be ordered by courts for remedial purposes (or implemented by means of consent decrees) (see Levin-Epstein 1987: Chapter 14).

12 Weale in fact refers to 'equality of benefit' but this is misleading insofar as it suggests 'equal benefits'. The principle requires *unequal* benefits to bring those with unequal needs to equality of welfare (see Weale 1978: 70).

13 In the present context this would entail different minority groups, not just the majority and all minority groups combined.

14 These questions also raise broader issues about the moral standing of groups for the purposes of compensation and distribution which will be considered in subsequent chapters, but see Thurow (1979), Sher (1981).

3 THE LOGIC OF AFFIRMATIVE ACTION

1 The implication that can be read into this argument, that it is possible (and desirable) to distinguish between harm or injury and the disadvantageous consequences that follow from it, is intended.

2 'Representation' is used here in a generic (and loose) sense. It is subject to a variety of interpretations which will be examined in subsequent pages.

3 The eight factors are given in an abbreviated form here; they are discussed in more detail in Chapter 5.

4 Sandel (1982: Chapter 2) has provided a useful commentary on, and critique of, Rawls's arguments here.

5 Whether we have such a right may depend on our preferred interpretation

of equality of opportunity. It may be thought that we have a right to compete fairly (without undue hindrance) but not to have the disadvantages of nature and nurture compensated for. The unelaborated idea of equal opportunity will suffice for present arguments however.

6 For a detailed legal critique of the content of this section of the Act, see Bindman (1979). This formulation of indirect discrimination is far from unproblematic but will suffice for the present for illustrative purposes.

7 For further discussion of this and the idea of 'reasonable business purpose' in the context of religion in Northern Ireland, see Standing Advisory Commission on Human Rights (1987: 60).

8 Possibly the best known case in Britain is *Raval v. Department of Health and Social Security and the Civil Service Commission* (Employment Appeals Tribunal 17.5.85) in which an 'O' Level English requirement for clerical posts in the Civil Service was found to have an adverse impact on applicants of Asian origin but also to be a genuine occupational qualification (see *Equal Opportunities Review* 1985b: 26–32).

4 AFFIRMATIVE ACTION IN EMPLOYMENT: THE BRITISH EXPERIENCE

1 Documentary sources are listed separately in the Bibliography on pp. 247–49.

2 This and the following account are based on City of A (1989d).

3 A formal equal opportunities statement had been in existence since 1982 however.

4 By 1991 the highest proportion in any plant was 40 per cent.

5 In practice, no equality targets are set for units in areas with no, or virtually no, ethnic minority population.

5 THE REAL THING: THE AMERICAN WAY WITH AFFIRMATIVE ACTION

1 Women were not yet to be included in these affirmative action programmes however.

2 For example: *United States v. Ironworkers* (1971), *Contractors Association v. Secretary of Labor* (1971).

3 The Wonderlic and Bennet Mechanical Aptitude Tests, which were professionally developed, and not in-house tests.

4 President Bush had already vetoed the 1990 Civil Rights Bill which had failed by one vote to gain the majority necessary to override the veto in Senate.

5 We shall be concerned here primarily with non-construction contractors. The requirements of construction contractors are slightly different (see EO 11246 Part III).

6 OFCCP is a part of the Employment Standards Administration which itself is a directorate of the Department of Labor (see Cooper 1987: 7–8).

7 Some parts of the RO4 details have been re-ordered in this account for the sake of brevity.

8 This is the name now conventionally given to this analysis though it is not called such in the Code of Federal Regulations.

9 This will be the same for many job titles, but for some (and especially senior positions) it will be different – and may even be state- or nation-wide.

10 This is a more detailed version of the list given in Chapter 3.

11 The '80 per cent rule' as used here is to be distinguished from the 'four-fifths rule' of adverse impact used in the validation of tests.
12 The process of test validation for non-discrimination and for a justification by virtue of 'business necessity' is further discussed in subsequent paragraphs.
13 As we have already noted, the 'business necessity' standard of validation was altered by the Supreme Court decision in *Ward's Cove Packing Co. v. Atonio* (1989) and then partially reinstated in the Civil Rights Act 1991.
14 A counter-argument to Blits and Gottfredson is to be found in Kelman (1990: 21).

6 RACE-CONSCIOUS PRACTICE: THE UNITED STATES

1 All these tests have been devised specifically for the W police force and have been continually monitored, analysed and validated by professional testers; see Morstain and Hsu (1977), Morstain (1988).
2 This is an argument that has a respectable (though not necessarily valid) pedigree; see for example Dworkin (1977a, 1977b, 1978).
3 This figure relates to 1991 and therefore does not coincide exactly with data in Table 6.3.
4 What this process of no-ranking within groups does is effectively to create a five-person 'tie-break', thus permitting the admission of non-'merit' criteria.
5 In 1987 72.4 per cent of whites who had been freshmen in 1984 returned for their fourth year compared with 59.9 per cent of black freshmen. Figures were better for the 1985 intake at 74.0 per cent and 67.3 per cent respectively. However, 51.1 per cent of 1984 white freshmen graduated in four years compared with only 31.3 per cent of blacks. Furthermore, the number of black freshmen in 1987 was *lower* than that in 1978 (134 and 140 respectively) (University of DU 1989d: Tables 1 and 2).
6 The *Ad Hoc* Committee that reviewed the university's Affirmative Action Plan made particular comparison with *The Madison Plan* of the University of Wisconsin at Madison (1988).

7 PRACTICE COMPARED: BRITAIN AND AMERICA

1 This is not to suggest that America is unique in this. Diversity has arrived in Britain but is not (yet) pursued with the same vigour.
2 This does not hold true for all sub-groups within the Asian category. Both Pakistani and Bangladeshi sub-groups remain among the most educationally deprived in Britain (see Brown 1984).
3 We need only look to the Houses of Commons and Lords for evidence of this habit as, for example, in the debates during the second reading of the Local Government Grants (Ethnic Groups) Bill in 1979 (*Hansard* 1979).
4 This finding in *Burdine* sits uneasily with the requirement laid upon contractors under EO 11246 to change employment practices where these are found to have a discriminatory impact.

8 THE MORAL DILEMMAS OF PREFERENCE

1 We have tidied up Fullinwider's argument here for the purposes of our own exposition – and omitted his subsequent disclaimer of rights to positions

on the grounds that beneficiaries are only instruments serving a larger purpose.

2 Consequentialism comes in a variety of forms; for a discussion of some of these, see Edwards (1987: Chapter 8).

3 We are not arguing here that race-conscious practices *are* so justified, only that deontic reasons are more compelling than consequential ones. I have discussed elsewhere the question of whether these practices are in fact justified (see Edwards 1987).

4 The argument has sometimes been made that there is a psychic benefit to be had by all members of a group by seeing another member succeed. A variant on this is the role model concept (see Thomson 1986, Exum 1983, O'Neil 1975, Bittker 1973, Boxhill 1977). Neither is convincing as the basis for policy intervention on any scale.

5 The term 'victim' is used here and throughout to mean 'someone who bears the costs'. 'Victim' has become closely associated with arguments against race-conscious practices. Its use here is for reasons of conciseness, not to imply sympathy with any particular view.

6 In *Wygant*, the Supreme Court found, by a 5–4 majority, that the Jackson Board of Education's collectively bargained lay-off plan in a school district to protect minority hiring gains violated the Fourteenth Amendment.

7 Lynch entitled his book *Invisible Victims: White Males and the Crisis of Affirmative Action* (1989).

8 The terms 'preference policy', 'preferred', etc. are used throughout this section. This is not meant to exclude affirmative action practices which, as we have already argued, are indistinguishable from preference at the margins.

9 Court-ordered remedies for egregious discrimination are an exception here.

10 Much turns on the idea of a 'fair competition' and we shall examine it in the next chapter.

11 Boxhill's argument is in fact stronger than at first appears. What he is calling for here (from beneficiary whites) is not just compensation for past harm but *reparation* for past wrong-doing.

12 Fiscus is silent on this. Although disallowing whites to compete for the 20 per cent of positions set aside for blacks there appears to be no equivalent proscription on blacks applying for the 80 per cent of white jobs.

13 This is Dworkin's argument in respect of *Bakke*; see Dworkin (1977, 1978).

14 Justice O'Connor also dissented over the question of whether the 50 per cent quota survived strict scrutiny (see Cathcart, Burcham and Sulds 1990: 10, Lively 1992: 138 ff.).

15 Boxhill was concerned with African-Americans in his argument; for the sake of the present discussion about generalities, we have extended it to all minority racial and ethnic groups.

16 Which is not to say that in the circumstances we are concerned with they have now been paid.

9 EQUAL OPPORTUNITIES, MERITS AND PREFERENCES

1 This distinction between the moral force of consequence-regarding and morally prescriptive actions follows the common differentiation between teleologic and deontic principles (see Frankena 1963, Finnis 1983, Hare 1978, Brandt 1979, Melden 1977).

2 The successful candidate may not be *the* best person for the job or *the* best

qualified for the job. There may be others better qualified who did not apply. The right attaches in virtue of being the best of the *applicants*.
3 This is only mildly irascible. We have illustrated in earlier chapters the somewhat baroque accounts that companies give in their justifications for the use of diversity. The bottom line, however, is almost always profit and competitiveness. After all, few companies are going to be prepared to carry the weight (and cost) of the 'rich cultural heritage that is diversity' if it consistently fails to deliver on what matters most.
4 We have to be careful in our formulation here and ought to qualify this statement at least to include only *legal* contributory factors.

10 TAILORED PREFERENCE

1 Particular techniques will of course differ as between employment practice and minority business set-asides.
2 Such statistical evaluations as have been undertaken have not produced a consensus of results, but the weight of evidence supports the view that affirmative action *has* produced significant gains for minorities (see Leonard 1984, 1985, Kellough 1989, Potomac Institute 1984, Office of Federal Contract Compliance Programs 1984, Organisation Resources Counselors 1984).
3 The percentage of employed people in the private sector who come from each racial or ethnic group.
4 Data extracted from United States Equal Employment Opportunity Commission (1989b).
5 These aggregated figures, however, mask some significant variations which highlight what was said earlier about the need for a more careful tailoring of race-conscious practice. Thus, for example, whilst the private sector participation rate for blacks increased from 8.2 per cent to 12.4 per cent between 1966 and 1988, the rate for black *males* remained almost static at 5.7 per cent and 5.9 per cent.
6 'Compensating' is here used in the sense of 'making up for wants', not as restitution for past harm.
7 I ended an earlier book with the opposite conclusion.

Bibliography

Abram, M. (1986) 'Affirmative Action: Fair Shakers and Social Engineers', *Harvard Law Review* 99 (6): 1312–46.

Alexander, L. (1990) 'Reconsidering the Relationship Among Voluntary Acts, Strict Liability, and Negligence in Criminal Law'. In E.F. Paul, F. Miller and J. Paul (eds) *Crime, Culpability, and Remedy*, Oxford: Blackwell.

Ansari, K. (1987) *Managing Britain's Multi-Racial Future: The Employment of Ethnic Minorities in Growth Industries in the Thames Valley*, Mimeo, The Management Centre, Slough College.

Anthony, W.P. and Bowen, M. (1977) 'Affirmative Action: Problems and Promises', *Personnel Journal* 56 (12): 616–21.

BACIE/Institute of Personnel Management (1987) *Be Fair: An Equal Opportunities Resource Manual*, London: Cabinet Office.

Ball, W and Solomos, J. (eds) (1990) *Race and Local Politics*, London: Macmillan.

Barry, B. (1965) *Political Argument*, London: Routledge and Kegan Paul.

Barry, B. (1967) 'Justice and the Common Good'. In A. Quinton (ed.) *Political Philosophy*, Oxford: Oxford University Press.

Bayles, M.D. (1973a) 'Compensatory Reverse Discrimination in Hiring', *Social Theory and Practice* 2 (3): 301–12.

Bayles, M.D. (1973b) 'Reparations to Wronged Groups', *Analysis* 33 (6): 182–84.

Belton, R. (1981) 'Discrimination and Affirmative Action: An Analysis of Competing Theories of Equality and '"Weber"', *North Carolina Law Review* 59 (1): 531–98.

Belz, H. (1991) *Equality Transformed: A Quarter-Century of Affirmative Action*, New York: Transaction Publishers.

Benn, S.I. and Peters, R.S. (1959) *Social Principles and the Democratic State*, London: Allen and Unwin.

Benyon, J. and Solomos, J. (eds) (1987) *The Roots of Urban Unrest*, Oxford: Pergamon Press.

Bindman, G. (1979) 'Indirect Discrimination and the Race Relations Act', *New Law Journal* 129 (5901): 408–11.

Bittker, B. (1973) *The Case for Black Reparations*, New York: Random House.

Blackstone, W.T. (1977) 'Reverse Discrimination and Compensatory Justice'. In W.T. Blackstone and R.D. Heslep (eds) *Social Justice and Preferential Treatment*, Athens: University of Georgia Press.

Blackstone, W.T. and Heslep, R.D. (eds) (1977) *Social Justice and Preferential Treatment*, Athens: University of Georgia Press.

Blits, J. and Gottfredson, L. (1990a) 'Employment Testing and Job Performance', *The Public Interest* No. 98, Winter: 18–25.

Blits, J. and Gottfredson, L. (1990b) 'Equality or Lasting Inequality?' *Society* March/April: 4.

Bolick, C. (1990) *Unfinished Business: A Civil Rights Strategy for America's Third Century*, Pacific Research Institute for Public Policy, Berkeley, Calif.

Bowser, W. (1989) *A Primer on Affirmative Action*, Mimeo, Wilmington, Del.: New Castle County Department of Law.

Bowser, W. (1990) *A Primer on Employment Discrimination Law*, Mimeo, Wilmington, Del.: New Castle County Department of Law.

Boxhill, B. (1977) 'The Morality of Reparation'. In B.R. Gross (ed.) *Reverse Discrimination*, Buffalo, N.Y.: Prometheus.

Braham, P., Rattansi, A. and Skellington, R. (eds) (1992) *Racism and Anti-Racism*, London: Sage.

Brandt, R.B. (1979) *A Theory of the Good and the Right*, Oxford: Oxford University Press.

Braybrooke, D. (1968) 'Let Needs Diminish That Preferences May Prosper', *American Philosophical Quarterly Monograph Series* 1: 86–107.

Braybrooke, D. (1987) *Meeting Needs*, Princeton: Princeton University Press.

Brown, C. (1984) *Black and White Britain: The Third Policy Studies Institute Survey*, London: Hutchinson.

Burney, E. (1988) *Steps to Racial Equality: Positive Action in a Negative Climate* (Runnymede Research Report), London: Runnymede Trust.

Campbell, T. (1988) *Justice*, London: Macmillan.

Capaldi, N. (1985) *Out of Order: Affirmative Action and the Crisis of Doctrinaire Liberalism*, Buffalo, N.Y.: Prometheus.

Carr, J. (1987) *New Roads to Equality: Contract Compliance for the UK?*, Fabian Society Tract No. 517, London: Fabian Society.

Carter, S. (1991) *Reflections of an Affirmative Action Baby*, New York: Basic Books.

Cathcart, D., Burcham, D. and Sulds, J. (1990) *Affirmative Action and Reverse Discrimination: Status of Quotas, Goals and the Emerging Standard of Strict Scrutiny*, Mimeo, Los Angeles: Gibson, Dunn and Crutcher.

Civil Rights Act (1964) Washington, D.C.

Civil Rights Act (1991) Washington, D.C. 51745.

Claiborne, L., Friedman, J., Cooke, B., Menon, K. and Stephen, D. (1983) *Race and Law in Britain and the United States*, London: Minority Rights Group.

Commission for Racial Equality (1980) *Guidance Note on Sikh Men and Women and Employment*, London: Commission for Racial Equality.

Commission for Racial Equality (1981a) *Commission for Racial Equality's Submission to Lord Scarman's Inquiry into Brixton Disorders*, London: Commission for Racial Equality.

Commission for Racial Equality (1981b) *In Search of a Skill: Ethnic Minority Youth and Apprenticeships*, London: Commission for Racial Equality.

Commission for Racial Equality (1982) *Further Education in a Multi-Racial Society: A Policy Report*, London: Commission for Racial Equality.

Commission for Racial Equality (1984) *Race Relations: Code of Practice*, London: Commission for Racial Equality.

Commission for Racial Equality (1985a) *Review of the Race Relations Act 1976: Proposals for Change*, London: Commission for Racial Equality.

Commission for Racial Equality (1985b) *Swann: A Response from the Commission for Racial Equality*, London: Commission for Racial Equality.

Commission for Racial Equality (1985c) *From Words to Action: Progress on the Race Relations Code of Practice. Employment Report Supplement*, London: Commission for Racial Equality.

Commission for Racial Equality (1987a) *Contract Compliance: Principles of Practice*, London: Commission for Racial Equality.

Commission for Racial Equality (1987b) *Comment on the Implications of the Local Government Bill,* London: Commission for Racial Equality.

Commission for Racial Equality (1989) *Are Employers Complying? A Research Report,* London: Commission for Racial Equality.

Confederation of British Industry (1981) 'Statement' and 'Guide on General Principles and Practice'. In P. Braham, E. Rhodes and M. Pearn (eds) *Discrimination and Disadvantage in Employment: The Experience of Black Workers,* London: Harper and Row.

Congressional Quarterly Almanac (1991) 'Compromise Civil Rights Bill Passed', *Congressional Quarterly Almanac* 1991: 251–61.

Congressional Quarterly Researcher (1991a) 'Racial Quotas: Can There Be Affirmative Action Without Special Preferences?' *Congressional Quarterly Researcher* 1 (2): 277–300.

Congressional Quarterly Researcher (1991b) 'Racial Quotas: Current Situation', *Congressional Quarterly Researcher* 1 (2): 290–94.

Cooper, J. (1987) *Affirmative Action and Equal Employment Opportunity Guide,* Washington, D.C.: J. Cooper and Associates Inc.

Cooper, M.H. (1991) 'Racial Questions', *Congressional Quarterly Researcher* 1 (2): 279–82.

Cowan, J.L. (1972) 'Inverse Discrimination', *Analysis* 33 (1): 10–12.

Cross, M. (1987a) *A Cause for Concern: Ethnic Minority Youth and Vocational Training Policy,* Warwick: Centre for Research in Ethnic Relations, University of Warwick.

Cross, M. (1987b) '"Equality of Opportunity" and Inequality of Outcome: The MSC, Ethnic Minorities and Training Policy'. In R. Jenkins and J. Solomos (eds) *Racism and Equal Opportunity Policies in the 1980s,* Cambridge: Cambridge University Press.

Day, J.P. (1981) 'Compensatory Discrimination', *Philosophy* 56 (1): 55–72.

Deakin, N. and Edwards, J. (1993) *The Enterprise Culture and the Inner City,* London: Routledge.

D'Souza, D. (1991) 'Sins of Admission', *The New Republic* 18 Feb: 30–35.

Dworkin, R. (1977a) *Taking Rights Seriously,* London: Duckworth.

Dworkin, R. (1977b) 'Why Bakke Has No Case', *New York Review of Books* 10 November: 11–15.

Dworkin, R. (1978) 'The Bakke Decision: Did it Decide Anything?' *New York Review of Books* 17 August: 20–25.

Dworkin, R. (1981) 'What is Equality? Part I: Equality of Welfare', *Philosophy and Public Affairs* 10 (3): 185–246.

Dwyer, P. (1989) 'The Blow to Affirmative Action May Not Hurt That Much', *Business Week* 3 July: 61.

Eastland, T. and Bennett, W. (1979) *Counting By Race: Equality from the Founding Fathers to Bakke and Weber,* New York: Basic Books.

Edwards, J. (1987) *Positive Discrimination, Social Justice and Social Policy,* London: Tavistock.

Edwards, J. (1988) 'Justice and the Bounds of Welfare', *Journal of Social Policy* 17 (2): 127–52.

Edwards, J. (1990a) 'What Purpose Does Equality of Opportunity Serve?' *New Community* 16 (2): 19–35.

Edwards, J. (1990b) *Affirmative Action and Preferential Treatment: An Evaluation of Costs and Benefits,* Newark: College of Urban Affairs and Public Policy, University of Delaware.

Edwards, J. (1990c) 'Affirmative Action "Culture" and US Equal Opportunity Practice', *Equal Opportunities Review* 34, November/December: 27–31.

Edwards, J. (1991) 'US Affirmative Action Alive and Well Despite Supreme Court', *Equal Opportunities International* 10 (1): 11–13.

Edwards, J. (1993) 'Gruppenrechte versus Individualrechte: Problem rassen und gruppenbezogener Politik', *Widersprüche* 46: 21–33.

Equal Employment Opportunity Commission (1986) *Title VII Enforces Job Rights*, Washington, D.C.: Equal Employment Opportunity Commission.

Equal Employment Opportunity Commission (1989a) *Equal Employment Opportunity: Standard Form 100 Rev.4–89, Employer Information Report E.E.O-1*, Washington, D.C.: Equal Employment Opportunity Commission.

Equal Employment Opportunity Commission (1989b) *Indicators of Equal Employment Opportunity: Status and Trends*, Washington, D.C.: Equal Employment Opportunity Commission.

Equal Opportunities Review (1985a) 'Racial Discrimination and Recruitment', *Equal Opportunities Review* No. 4, November/December: 19.

Equal Opportunities Review (1985b) 'English Language Discrimination Claim Fails: Raval v. Department of Health and Social Security and The Civil Service Commission', *Equal Opportunities Review* No. 3, September–October: 26–32.

Equal Opportunities Review (1987) 'Achieving Equal Opportunity Through Positive Action', *Equal Opportunities Review* No. 14, July/August: 13–17.

Equal Opportunities Review (1989a) 'Working for Race Equality at Leicester City Council', *Equal Opportunities Review* No. 25, May/June: 15–20.

Equal Opportunities Review (1989b) 'Equal Opportunity at Ford Motor Company', *Equal Opportunities Review* No. 24, March/April: 9–12.

Equal Opportunities Review (1989c) 'US Supreme Court Rulings Erode Equal Opportunities', *Equal Opportunities Review* No. 28, November/December: 23–25.

Exum, W.H. (1983) 'Climbing the Crystal Stair: Values, Affirmative Action and Minority Faculty', *Social Problems* 30 (4): 383–99.

Feinberg, J. (1973) *Social Philosophy*, Englewood Cliffs: Prentice Hall.

Feinberg, J. (1980) *Rights, Justice, and the Bounds of Liberty*, Princeton: Princeton University Press.

Feinberg, J. (1986) 'Wrongful Life and the Counterfactual Element in Harming', *Social Philosophy and Policy* 4 (1): 145–78.

Finnis, J. (1983) *Fundamentals of Ethics*, Oxford: Clarendon Press.

Fiscus, R. (1992) *The Constitutional Logic of Affirmative Action*, Durham: Duke University Press.

Fishkin, J.A. (1987) 'Liberty Versus Equal Opportunity', *Social Philosophy and Policy* 5 (1): 32–48.

Flaugher, R. (1977) *The Many Definitions of Test Bias*, Research Memorandum 77–2, Princeton: Educational Testing Service.

Frankena, W.K. (1962) 'The Concept of Social Justice'. In R.B. Brandt (ed.) *Social Justice*, Englewood Cliffs: Prentice Hall.

Frankena, W.K. (1963) *Ethics*, Englewood Cliffs: Prentice Hall.

Fried, C. (1978) *Right and Wrong*, Cambridge, Mass.: Harvard University Press.

Fullinwider, R.K. (1980) *The Reverse Discrimination Controversy*, Totowa, N.J.: Rowman and Littlefield.

Fullinwider, R.K. (1986) 'Reverse Discrimination and Equal Opportunity'. In J.P. De Marco and R.M. Fox (eds) *New Directions in Ethics: The Challenge of Applied Ethics*, London: Routledge and Kegan Paul.

Glazer, N. (1975) *Affirmative Discrimination, Ethnic Inequality and Public Policy*, New York: Basic Books.

Goldman, A. (1975) 'Reparations to Individuals or Groups?' *Analysis* 35: 168–70.

Goldman, A. (1976) 'Affirmative Action', *Philosophy and Public Affairs* 5 (2): 178–95.

Goldman, A. (1977) 'Affirmative Action'. In M. Cohen, T. Nagel and T. Scanlon (eds) *Equality and Preferential Treatment*, Princeton: Princeton University Press.

Goldman, A. (1979) *Justice and Reverse Discrimination*, Princeton: Princeton University Press.

Goldman, A. (1987) 'The Justification of Equal Opportunity', *Social Philosophy and Policy* 5 (1): 88–103.

Goldstein, B. (1989) 'New Civil Rights Legislation Essential', Washington, D.C.: Daily Labor Report.

Greater London Enterprise Board (1985) *Redressing the Balance: Backing Black Enterprise in London*, London: Greater London Enterprise Board.

Greene, M. (1977) 'Equality and Inviolability: An Approach to Compensatory Justice'. In W.T. Blackstone and R.D. Heslep (eds) *Social Justice and Preferential Treatment*, Athens: University of Georgia Press.

Gross, B.R. (ed.) (1977) *Reverse Discrimination*, Buffalo, N.Y.: Prometheus Books.

Gross, B.R. (1978) *Discrimination in Reverse*, New York: New York University Press.

Gross, B.R. (1987) 'Real Equality of Opportunity', *Social Philosophy and Policy* 5 (1): 120–42.

Guttman, A. (1980) *Liberal Equality*, Cambridge: Cambridge University Press.

Hacker, A. (1989) 'Affirmative Action: The New Look', *The New York Review* 12 October: 63–68.

Hansard (1979) House of Commons, 12 March, cols 78 et seq. (Debate on Local Government Grants (Ethnic Groups) Bill).

Hare, R.M. (1978) 'Justice and Equality'. In J. Arthur and W.H. Shaw (eds) *Justice and Economic Distribution*, Englewood Cliffs: Prentice Hall.

Hartigan, J. and Wigdor, A. (eds) (1989) *Fairness in Employment Testing: Validity Generalisation, Minority Issues, and the General Aptitude Test Battery*, Washington, D.C.: National Academy of Sciences.

Helm, S. (1987) '"Second Chance" Plan to Recruit More Black Police', *Independent* 16 June.

Higgins, J. (1978) *The Poverty Business: Britain and America*, Oxford: Blackwell.

Hoffman, R. (1977) 'Justice, Merit, and the Good'. In B.R. Gross (ed.) *Reverse Discrimination*, Buffalo, N.Y.: Prometheus Books.

Home Office (1977) *Racial Discrimination: A Guide to the Race Relations Act 1976*, London: HMSO.

Honoré, A.M. (1968) 'Social Justice'. In R.S. Summers (ed.) *Essays in Legal Philosophy*, Oxford: Blackwell.

House of Commons (1981) Home Affairs Committee: Race Relations and Immigration Sub-Committee: Session 1980–81, Fifth Report, *Racial Disadvantage*, H.C. 424 IV, London: HMSO.

House of Commons (1982) Home Affairs Select Committee: Fifth Report: *Racial Disadvantage*, Session 1980–81: *The Government Reply*. Cmnd. 8476, London: HMSO.

House of Commons (1987a) House of Commons Employment Committee: First Report: *Discrimination in Employment*, H.C. 180, London: HMSO.

House of Commons (1987b) House of Commons Employment Committee: *Discrimination in Employment: Memoranda Laid Before the Committee*, London: HMSO.

Hudson Institute (1987) *Workforce 2000: Work and Workers for the 21st Century*, Indianapolis: Hudson Institute.

Hudson Institute (1988) *Opportunity 2000: Creative Affirmative Action Strategies for a Changing Workforce*, Washington, D.C.: US Department of Labor.

Inner London Education Authority (1986) *Contract Compliance in the Community,* London: ILEA.

Institute of Personnel Management (1986) *The Institute of Personnel Management Equal Opportunities Code,* London: Institute of Personnel Management.

Institute of Personnel Management (1987a) *Contract Compliance: The UK Experience,* London: Institute of Personnel Management.

Institute of Personnel Management (1987b) 'Contract Compliance: Can We Learn from the States?', *Institute of Personnel Management Digest* No. 263, June 1987: 15–16.

Kellough, J. (1989) *Federal Equal Employment Opportunity Policy and Numerical Goals and Timetables,* New York: Praeger.

Kelman, M. (1990) 'The Problem of False Negatives', *Society* March/April: 21.

Kennedy, R. (1986) 'Persuasion and Distrust: A Comment on the Affirmative Action Debate', *Harvard Law Review* 99 (6): 1327–45.

Killian, L. (1990) 'Redressive Action and Ethnic Relations in the United States'. In S.K. Mitra (ed.) *Politics of Positive Discrimination,* London: Sangam Books.

King's Fund (1987) *A Model Policy for Equal Opportunities in Employment in the National Health Service,* Equal Opportunities Task Force, Occasional Paper No. 1, London: King's Fund.

Kirp, D. and Weston, N. (1987) 'The Political Jurisprudence of Affirmative Action', *Social Philosophy and Policy* 5 (1): 223–48.

Leonard, J. (1984) *The Impact of Affirmative Action,* Washington, D.C.: US Department of Labor.

Leonard, J. (1985) 'What Promises are Worth: The Impact of Affirmative Action Goals', *Journal of Human Resources* 20 (1): 3–20.

Levin-Epstein, M.D. (1987) *Primer of Equal Employment Opportunity* (4th edn), Washington, D.C.: Bureau of National Affairs Inc.

Lively, D. (1992) *The Constitution and Race,* New York: Praeger.

Local Government Act (1988), London: HMSO.

Loury, G.C. (1987) 'Why Should We Care About Group Inequality?' *Social Philosophy and Policy* 5 (1): 249–75.

Lucas, J.R. (1980) *On Justice,* Oxford: Clarendon Press.

Lustgarten, L. and Edwards, J. (1992) 'Racial Inequality and the Limits of the Law'. In P. Braham, A. Rattansi and R. Skellington (eds) *Racism and Anti-Racism,* London: Sage.

Lynch, F. (1989) *Invisible Victims: White Males and the Crisis of Affirmative Action,* New York: Greenwood Press.

McCrudden, C., Smith, D. and Brown, C. (1991) *Racial Justice at Work,* London: Policy Studies Institute.

Marris, P. and Rein, M. (1967) *Dilemmas of Social Reform,* Harmondsworth: Penguin.

Melden, A.I. (1977) *Rights and Persons,* Oxford: Blackwell.

Miller, D. (1976) *Social Justice,* Oxford: Clarendon Press.

Mishkin, P.J. (1983) 'The Uses of Ambivalence: Reflections on the Supreme Court and the Constitutionality of Affirmative Action', *University of Pennsylvania Law Review* 131 (4): 907–31.

Mitra, S.K. (ed.) (1990) *Politics of Positive Discrimination,* London: Sangam Books.

Morstain, B. (1988) *The 1987 Promotion System for the Wilmington Department of Police,* Newark: College of Urban Affairs and Public Policy, University of Delaware.

Morstain, B. and Hsu, L. (1977) *Delaware Co-operative Police Selection Study. Test*

Validation Study: Technical Report, Newark: College of Urban Affairs and Public Policy, University of Delaware.

Moynihan, D.P. (1969) *Maximum Feasible Misunderstanding*, New York: The Free Press.

Murphy, W. (1989) *Supreme Court Review* (Mimeo) (Paper presented at Annual Meeting ABA Labor and Employment Law Section).

Nagel, T. (1977) 'Equal Treatment and Compensatory Justice'. In M. Cohen, T. Nagel and T. Scanlon (eds) *Equality and Preferential Treatment*, Princeton: Princeton University Press.

Nakanishi, D. (1989) 'A Quota on Excellence: The Asian American Admissions Debate', *Change* November/December: 39.

Nickel, J.W. (1972) 'Discrimination and Morally Relevant Characteristics', *Analysis* 32 (4): 113–14.

Nickel, J.W. (1973) 'Should Reparations Be to Individuals or Groups?' *Analysis* 34 (5): 154–60.

Nickel, J.W. (1977) 'Preferential Policies in Hiring and Admissions: A Jurisprudential Approach'. In B. Gross (ed.) *Reverse Discrimination*, Buffalo, N.Y.: Prometheus Books.

Nunn, W.A. (1973) 'Reverse Discrimination', *Analysis* 34 (5): 151–54.

Oakley, R. (1988) *Employment in Police Forces: A Survey of Equal Opportunities*, London: Commission for Racial Equality.

Office of Federal Contract Compliance Programs (1984) *Employment Patterns of Minorities and Women in Federal Contractor and Non-Contractor Establishments 1974–80*, Washington, D.C.: Department of Labor.

Office of Federal Contract Compliance Programs (1987) *Making Equal Employment Opportunity Work*, Washington, D.C.: Department of Labor.

O'Neil, O. (1987) 'Rights to Compensation', *Social Philosophy and Policy* 5 (1): 72–87.

O'Neil, R.M. (1975) *Discriminating Against Discrimination*, Bloomington: Indiana University Press.

O'Neill, J.E. (1987) 'Discrimination and Income Inequality', *Social Philosophy and Policy* 5 (1): 169–87.

Organisation Resources Counselors Inc. (1984) *Managing Diversity: The Challenge of Equal Employment Opportunity to 1990*, New York: Organisation Resources Counselors Inc.

Pearn, M. (1978) *Employment Testing and the Goal of Equal Opportunity: The American Experience*, London: Runnymede Trust.

Perelman, C. (1963) *The Idea of Justice and the Problem of Argument*, New York: Humanities Press.

Personnel Management (1990) 'Police in Drive to Attract More Black Recruits', *Personnel Management* March: 91.

Plowden Report (1967) *Report of the Central Advisory Committee for Education: Children and Their Primary Schools*, London: HMSO.

Potomac Institute Inc. (1984) *A Decade of New Opportunity: Affirmative Action in the 1970s*, Washington, D.C.: Potomac Institute.

Presidential Executive Order 8802 (1941), Washington, D.C.: Government Printing Office.

Presidential Executive Order 10925 (1961), Washington, D.C.: Government Printing Office.

Presidential Executive Order 11246 (1965), Washington, D.C.: Government Printing Office.

Presidential Executive Order 11375 (1967), Washington, D.C.: Government Printing Office.

Presidential Executive Order 12067 (1978), Washington, D.C.: Government Printing Office.

Presidential Executive Order 12086 (1978), Washington, D.C.: Government Printing Office.

Race Relations Act (Great Britain) (1976), London: HMSO.

Raphael, D.D. (1976) *Problems of Political Philosophy*, London: Macmillan.

Rawls, J. (1972) *A Theory of Justice*, Oxford: Oxford University Press.

Rescher, N. (1966) *Distributive Justice*, Indianapolis: Bobbs-Merrill.

Rex, J. (1988) *The Ghetto and the Underclass*, Aldershot: Avebury.

Rosenberg, A. (1987) 'The Political Philosophy of Biological Endowments: Some Considerations', *Social Philosophy and Policy* 5 (1): 1–31.

Ross, A. (1974) *On Law and Justice*, London: Stevens.

Ruzicho, A.J. (1980) 'The Weber Case – Its Impact on Affirmative Action', *Personnel Administrator* 25 (6): 69–72.

St Antoine, T. (1989) *Presentation to Southwestern Legal Foundation's 36th Annual Institute on Labor Law in Dallas* (Untitled) Washington, D.C.: Bureau of National Affairs Inc.

Sandel, M. (1982) *Liberalism and the Limits of Justice*, Cambridge: Cambridge University Press.

Sher, G. (1977) 'Justifying Reverse Discrimination in Employment'. In M.Cohen, T. Nagel and T. Scanlon (eds) *Equality and Preferential Treatment*, Princeton: Princeton University Press.

Sher, G. (1981) 'Ancient Wrongs and Modern Rights', *Philosophy and Public Affairs* 10 (1): 3–17.

Sher, G. (1987) 'Predicting Performance', *Social Philosophy and Policy* 5 (1): 188–203.

Shiner, R.A. (1973) 'Individuals, Groups and Inverse Discrimination', *Analysis* 33 (6): 185–87.

Silvestri, P. (1973) 'The Justification of Inverse Discriminaton', *Analysis* 34 (1): 31.

Simon, R. (1977) 'Preferential Hiring: A Reply to Judith Jarvis Thomson'. In M. Cohen, T. Nagel and T. Scanlon (eds) *Equality and Preferential Treatment*, Princeton: Princeton University Press.

Singer, P. (1979) *Practical Ethics*, Cambridge: Cambridge University Press.

Skerry, P. (1989) 'Immigration and the Affirmative Action State', *The Public Interest* 96 (Summer): 86–102.

Smith, D.J. (1977) *Racial Disadvantage in Britain*, Harmondsworth: Penguin.

Smith, J. and Welch, F. (1986) *Closing the Gap: Forty Years of Economic Progress for Blacks*, Washington D.C.: The Rand Corporation.

Sowell, T. (1975) 'Affirmative Action Reconsidered: Was it Necessary in Academia?' *Evaluative Studies* 27: 5–6 (American Enterprise Institute).

Sowell, T. (1977) '"Affirmative Action" Reconsidered'. In B.G. Gross (ed.) *Reverse Discrimination*, Buffalo, N.Y.: Prometheus Books.

Sowell, T. (1990) *Preferential Policies: An International Perspective*, New York: William Morrow.

Standing Advisory Commission on Human Rights (1987) *Religious and Political Discrimination and Equality of Opportunity in Northern Ireland: Report on Fair Employment*. Cm. 237, Belfast: HMSO.

Steele, S. (1990a) 'A Negative Vote on Affirmative Action', *New York Times Magazine* 13 May: 47 et seq.

Steele , S. (1990b) *The Content of Our Character*, New York: St Martin's Press.

Steiner, H. (1987) 'Capitalism, Justice and Equal Starts', *Social Philosophy and Policy* 5 (1): 49–71.

Swann (1985) Department of Education and Science: *Education for All: Committee of Inquiry into the Education of Children from Ethnic Minority Groups* (The Swann Report) Cmnd. 9453, London: HMSO.

Taylor, P.W. (1973) 'Reverse Discrimination and Compensatory Justice', *Analysis* 33 (6): 177–82.

Thomas, C. (1982) *Luncheon Address: FBA/BNA Fifth Annual Conference on Equal Employment Opportunity,* Washington, D.C.: Mimeo.

Thomson, J.J. (1986) *Rights, Restitution and Risk: Essays in Moral Theory,* Cambridge, Mass.: Harvard University Press.

Thurow, L. (1979) 'A Theory of Groups and Economic Redistribution', *Philosophy and Public Affairs* 9 (1): 25–41.

Timmins, N. (1982) 'Extra Training Urged to Get More Black Police', *The Times* 27 July.

Uniform Guidelines (USA) (1974) *Uniform Guidelines on Employment Selection Procedures*: 401 FEP Manual 2231.

United States Code (1976) 42 United States Code Section 2000d M.

United States Code of Federal Regulations (1985) 29 Code of Federal Regulations Chapter XIV, Washington, D.C.

United States Code of Federal Regulations (1989) *41 Code of Federal Regulations Chapter 60* – Office of Federal Contract Compliance Programs, Equal Employment Opportunity, Department of Labor, Washington, D.C.

United States Law Week (1989) 'Ward's Cove Packing Co. v. Atonio', *United States Law Week* 57 LW 4588.

University of Madison-Wisconsin (1988) *The Madison Plan.*

Van Alstyne, W. (1979) 'Rites of Passage: Race, the Supreme Court, and the Constitution', *University of Chicago Review* 46 (4): 775–810.

Vlastos, G. (1962) 'Justice and Equality'. In R.B. Brandt (ed.) *Social Justice,* Englewood Cliffs: Prentice Hall.

Von Leyden, W (1963) 'On Justifying Inequality', *Political Studies* 11 (1): 56–70.

Walzer, M. (1983) *Spheres of Justice: A Defence of Pluralism and Equality,* Oxford: Blackwell.

Weale, A. (1978) *Equality and Social Policy,* London: Routledge and Kegan Paul.

Williams, B. (1962) 'The Idea of Equality'. In P. Laslett and D. Runciman (eds) *Philosophy, Politics and Society* 2nd series, London: Blackwell.

Williams, B. (1969) 'The Idea of Equality'. In J. Feinberg (ed.) *Moral Concepts,* Oxford: Oxford University Press.

Wrench, J. (1986) *Unequal Comrades: Trade Unions, Equal Opportunity and Racism* (Policy Paper in Ethnic Relations, No. 5), Centre for Research in Ethnic Relations, University of Warwick.

UNITED STATES CASES CITED

Albermarle Paper Co. v. Moody 422 US 405 (1975).

City of Richmond v. J.A. Croson Co. 488 US 469 (1989).

Contractors Association v. Secretary of Labour 442F. 2d 153 (Third Circuit) 404 US 854 (1971).

Davis v. County of Los Angeles 13 FEP Cases 1217; 16 FEP Cases 396 45 91 (1976).

Dothard v. Rawlinson 433 US 321, 15 FEP Cases 10 29 91 (1977).

Equal Employment Opportunity Commission Decision No. 71–797, 3 FEP Cases 266–91 (1971).

Equal Employment Opportunity Commission Decision No. 72–0427, 4 FEP Cases 304 91 (1972).

Firefighters Local 1785 v. Stotts 467 US 561 (1984).

Franks v. Bowman Transportation Co. 424 US 747 (1976).

Green v. Missouri Pacific Railroad 523 F2d 1290, 1 FEP cases 1409 90 (1975).
Gregory v. Litton Systems Inc. 472 F2d 631, 5 FEP Cases 267 90 (1972).
Griggs v. Duke Power 401 US 424 (1971).
Independent Federation of Flight Attendants v. Zipes 491 US 754 (1989).
Local 28 Sheet Metal Workers v. Equal Employment Opportunity Commission 478 US 421 (1986).
Local 93 of the International Association of Firefighters v. City of Cleveland 478 US 501 (1986).
Lorance v. AT & T Technologies 490 US 900 (1989).
Martin v. Wilks 490 US 755 (1989).
New York City Transit Authority v. Beazer 440 US 568 (1979).
Patterson v. McLean Credit Union 491 US 164 (1989).
Price Waterhouse v. Hopkins 490 US 228 (1989).
Regents of the University of California v. Bakke 438 US 265 (1978).
Teamsters v. United States 431 US 324 (1977).
Texas Department of Community Affairs v. Burdine 450 US 248 (1981).
United States v. Georgia Power 474 F2d 906, 5 FEP Cases 587 90 (1973).
United States v. Ironworkers 86 443F. 2d 544 (Ninth Circuit), 404 US 984 (1971).
United States v. Paradise 480 US 149 (1987).
United Steelworkers v. Weber 443 US 193 (1979).
Ward's Cove Packing Co. v. Atonio 490 US 642 (1989).
Washington v. Davis 426 US 229 (1976).
Wygant v. Jackson Board of Education 476 US 106 (1986).

DOCUMENTARY SOURCES

City of A (1988a) *The Future Population of A: 1988 Review: Summary Statement*, Race Relations Advisory Group.
City of A (1988b) *Employee Audit Headcount 1987*, Directorate of Personnel.
City of A (1989a) *Race Relations: A Model for Action*, Chief Executive and Policy Development Officers (Race Relations Policy Statement).
City of A (1989b) *Action for Excellence: The Strategic Plan 1989/90 and Beyond*.
City of A (1989c) *A Model for the 1990s*, Policy and Resources Committee.
City of A (1989d) *Race Relations Profile and Action Plan 1989/90*, Directorate of Finance: Report to the Policy and Resources Support Services Sub-Committee.
City of A (undated) *Community Forums: Council Document*.
London Borough of B (1986) *Report on Racial/Gender Monitoring Statistics*, Staffing and Equal Opportunities Committee.
London Borough of B (1987a) *Towards Equality: Equal Employment Opportunities Policy and Programme of Action*.
London Borough of B (1987b) *Introduction to the Equal Opportunities Policy*.
London Borough of B (1987c) *Equal Opportunities Statement*.
London Borough of B (1989) *Report on Racial/Gender Composition of the Council's Workforce*, Race Relations Committee, Staffing and Equal Opportunities Committee and Women's Committee.
London Borough of B (1990) *Equal Opportunities and Community Affairs*, Report to the Policy and Resources Committee.
C County Council (1988) *Equal Opportunities Headcount Survey*.
C County Council (1989a) *C County Council – Equality Objectives*, Report of the Clerk of the Council and Chief Executive to the Resources Committee.
C County Council (1989b) *Equal Opportunities – Recruitment and Selection Monitoring*, Report of the Acting County Personnel Officer.

C County Council (1990) *Equal Opportunities – Recruitment and Selection Monitoring*, Report of the Acting County Personnel Officer.

D City Council (1982) *The Council's Policy on Equal Opportunity in Employment.*

D City Council (1986) *Monitoring of Employment Statistics*, Report of the Director of Personnel and Management Services.

D City Council (1988) *Monitoring of Employment Statistics*, Report of the Director of Personnel and Management Services.

D City Council (1989) *Positive Action (Race Relations) Annual Report*, Report of the Chief Executive to the Policy and Resources (Equal Opportunities) Sub-Committee and the Policy and Resources Committee.

E County Council (1987) *Equal Opportunities and Race Relations Department.*

E County Council (1988) *Recruitment and Selection: Personnel Procedures Handbook*, County Personnel Department.

F City Council (1988) *Code of Practice in Recruitment and Selection.*

F City Council (1989a) *Annual Report 1988/89: Ethnic Minorities Advisory Committee.*

F City Council (1989b) *Report of the Director of Administration, Staff Audit.*

F City Council (1990) *Developing a Strategic Approach to Equality Issues in F*, Department of Administration.

JX Bank (1989) *Equal Opportunities in JX.*

JX Bank (1990a) *Managing People Fairly: Equal Opportunities Training for Line Managers: Leaders Guide*, JX Personnel Department.

JX Bank (1990b) *Equal Opportunities – Progress Report and Recommendations for 1990: Report to the Personnel Committee of the Board*, Equal Opportunities Manager.

KX Company (1970) *KX of Britain: Race Relations Policy*, Central Labour Relations.

KX Company (1988) *KX of Britain Joint Statement on Equal Opportunity*, Personnel Department.

KX Company (1989) *1988 Equal Opportunities Report*, Equal Opportunities Department.

LX Airline (1978) *LX Policy on Racial Discrimination*, Group Instruction No. 68, 27 June.

LX Airline (1984a) *LX Equal Opportunity in Employment*, Standing Instruction No. 7.

LX Airline (1984b) *LX Human Resources Strategy Board.*

LX Airline (1985) *LX Racial Discrimination: Employment Policy and Procedure: Memorandum No. CS-10*, Human Resources Department.

LX Airline (1989) *Ethnic Minorities: Internal Memorandum.*

Industrial Relations Review and Report 202 (1979), June.

MX Organisation (1986) *Equal Opportunities Code of Practice.*

MX Organisation (1987) *The MX Organisation, Equal Opportunities and Race Equality: Five-Year Plan 1987–1992.*

MX Organisation (1989a) *Equal Opportunities.*

MX Organisation (1989b) *The MX Organisation – Recruitment – Equal Opportunities.*

Equal Employment Opportunity Commission (1972) *Equal Employment Opportunity Report 1970: Job Patterns for Minorities and Women in Private Industry Vol. 1*, Washington, D.C.: Equal Employment Opportunity Commission.

Equal Employment Opportunity Commission (1981) *Equal Employment Opportunity Commission 1979 Report: Minorities and Women in Private Industry Vol. 1*, Washington, D.C.: Equal Employment Opportunity Commission.

City of W (1990a) *Workforce Analysis 1984 and 1988.*

City of W (1990b) *Equal Opportunity Affirmative Action Plan 1990.*

City of W (1990c) *Equal Employment Opportunity: Policy Statement.*

City of W (1990d) *Affirmative Action Program.*

City of W Office of Public Safety (1990) *Department of Police: Monthly Report,* January.

State of D (1986) *Executive Order Number Twenty-Four: Affirmative Action in State Employment.*

State of D (1987) *Merit Rules: Rules for a Merit System of Personnel Administration.*

State of D (1989a) *Workforce Analysis 1989.*

State of D (1989b) *D Affirmative Action Program Notice: Policy Statement.*

State of D (1990) *Action Steps to Equal Employment Opportunity/Affirmative Action Advisory Council Report,* State Personnel Office.

University of DU (1986) *Equal Employment Opportunity and Affirmative Action Program.*

University of DU (1989a) *The University of DU: Facts and Figures: 1989–90.*

University of DU (1989b) *Equal Employment Opportunity and Affirmative Action Program.*

University of DU (1989c) *An Overview of the University of DU's Affirmative Action Commitment.*

University of DU (1989d) *A Report of the All University Committee on the Retention of Black Students.*

University of DU (1989e) *Report of the President's Commission to Promote Racial and Cultural Diversity.*

University of DU (1990) *Report of the Ad Hoc Committee to Review the Affirmative Action Plan.*

University of DU (undated) *Affirmative Action Recruitment Manual.*

SA Company (1989) *Diversity: A Source of Strength.*

Name index

Subject index